To PB

c̄ deep appreciation

Bill Anlyan

April 10/73

The future of medical education

The future of medical education

William G. Anlyan, M.D.

W. Gerald Austen, M.D.

John C. Beck, M.D.

William D. Bradford, M.D.

Ray E. Brown

Martin Cherkasky, M.D.

Lloyd C. Elam, M.D.

Thomas D. Kinney, M.D.

Irving M. London, M.D.

Donald N. Medearis, Jr., M.D.

Eugene A. Stead, Jr., M.D.

William G. Van der Kloot, Ph.D.

Judy Graves, *coordinating editor*

Duke University Press
Durham, N.C.
1973

© 1973, Duke University Press

L.C.C. card no. 72–97153

I.S.B.N. 0–8223–0294–2

Printed in the United States of America
by Kingsport Press, Inc.

Contents

Contributors

William G. Anlyan, M.D., Vice President for Health Affairs, Duke University Medical Center.

W. Gerald Austen, M.D., Professor of Surgery, Harvard Medical School; Chief of the Surgical Services, Massachusetts General Hospital.

John C. Beck, M.D., Professor and Chairman, Department of Medicine, McGill University; Physician-In-Chief, Royal Victoria Hospital.

William D. Bradford, M.D., Associate Professor of Pathology, Duke University Medical Center.

Ray E. Brown, Executive Vice President, Northwestern University, McGaw Medical Center.

Martin Cherkasky, M.D., Director, Montefiore Hospital and Medical Center; Atran Professor of Social Medicine, Albert Einstein College of Medicine.

Lloyd C. Elam, M.D., President, Meharry Medical College.

Thomas D. Kinney, M.D., Director of Medical and Allied Health Education; Professor and Chairman, Department of Pathology, Duke University Medical Center.

Irving M. London, M.D., Professor of Biology, Massachusetts Institute of Technology; Visiting Professor of Medicine, Harvard Medical School; Director of Harvard-M.I.T. Program in Health Sciences and Technology.

Donald N. Medearis, Jr., M.D., Dean, School of Medicine, University of Pittsburgh.

Eugene A. Stead, Jr., M.D., Professor of Medicine, Duke University Medical Center.

William G. Van der Kloot, Ph.D., Professor and Chairman, Department of Physiology and Biophysics, Health Sciences Center, State University of New York at Stony Brook.

Recommendations

1. Before the end of this decade, good quality care should be universally guaranteed by federal statute to every American—not merely planned and financed, but *guaranteed.*

2. The responsibility for making the benefits of the health care system equally available to everyone should be shared by all Americans. It is important, therefore, to initiate active recruitment and financial support of future doctors and other health professionals from all segments of the population.

3. Medical education should be designed as a true continuum extending from secondary school through college, medical school, hospital training, and postgraduate education. The concept of a continuum should be extended to the education of all health professionals, and all such educational programs should take place within the framework of the university.

4. An expanded curriculum in human biology should constitute the basis for the continuum of medical education. Its interfaces with the other natural sciences and with the social and behavioral sciences should be developed through multidisciplinary educational and research efforts. These programs should be designed to produce physicians and other health professionals for actual delivery of health services and also scientists and educators for research and teaching in the health sciences.

5. Because medical research has brought about vast improvements in health care and has more than paid for itself through savings in medical costs and human productivity, the funding for research and for the training of investigators in all of the sciences allied to medicine should be substantially expanded. The level should reflect both high national aspirations and a reasoned estimate of sums that can be used effectively.

6. Periodic recertification of physicians and a system of incentives for continuing education must be introduced as mechanisms for insuring the maintenance of a high level of professional competence. Techniques should include a review of physician performance using newer patient data storage systems and the other new evaluation methods for testing qualities essential to clinical competence. The development and implementation of such techniques fall within the responsibility of the university in consultation with appropriate professional and government agencies. The fiscal and human resources to achieve these ends must be made available.

7. The federal government should accept ultimate major responsibility for financing medical education. This responsibility should be clearly outlined, fixed and accepted, and should include the cost of both facilities and student aid.

8. Graduate medical education should become the responsibility of the university and the faculty of the medical center and not left solely to individual departments.

9. The graduate education of physicians should be designed to produce specialists and skills as required by the health care delivery system under which they will work. A time-availability system is suggested as a basis on which to plan residency programs for physicians and training of non-physician health personnel.

10. Universities as well as their medical schools should be responsive to the constantly changing health needs of society. They should help their communities and the nation develop workable models of health care and should initiate imaginative and diverse curricula and methods for the education of physicians and allied health personnel.

11. American medical schools must strive responsibly to exercise their unparalleled freedom to experiment for the improvement of medical education. With few restraints other than their own judgment, faculties can now revise curricula, shift goals, or modify admissions criteria to meet changing needs. In an era when government must take increasing responsibility for health education and care, this most valuable asset of freedom must be carefully safeguarded.

12. By 1985, the United States should be able to produce 25,000 new physicians each year. This will require maximum use of facilities and faculties, adequate financing, shortened and innovative curricula, and a modest number of new medical schools.

Foreword

It all started at the end of September 1971. Bill Anlyan, with whom I served as Visiting Professor of Medical Education at Duke University, took me to New York for two days to attend a meeting of outstanding medical educators who had gathered to revise the final draft of their collective volume, *The Future of Medical Education.* As an invited bystander, I promised myself that I would listen and keep quiet.

During several hours of stimulating discussions, I was deeply impressed by the stringent self-criticism to which the members of the group were willing to submit themselves. Almost every facet of American medical education was spread out on the dissection table, stripped, and examined with much disappointment and sorrow. At a given moment, I felt as though I were attending a masochistic seance. Finally, the compulsion to speak out overcame my determination to remain silent. Coming from a distant country where one is constantly reminded that "there is no prophet in his own city," and having the advantage of being far from home, I told my colleagues that they were exaggerating. With all my admiration for their spirit of constructive self-criticism, I felt compelled to remind them that by international standards, there is probably no second to American medical education, regardless of all of its shortcomings and its occasional failures. If freedom, flexibility, and experimentation are the main prerequisites for progress, there is no other place in the world where all three have been so consistently and fruitfully applied to promoting new approaches, exploring new techniques, and trying new concepts. The academic freedom of American medical faculties and the maturity of their students have been the sources of invaluable experience and innovations which have made the United States a leading force for progress in scientific medicine and medical education. I told my colleagues that the very fact that twelve outstanding medical scientists had decided to examine medical education in the past and to direct their efforts toward molding its future by writing such a book is, in itself, the most conclusive proof of American leadership. I probably sounded sincere and quite emotional. In any case, a few days later Bill Anlyan told me that the coauthors would like me to write a foreword to their book. It is a genuine honor and privilege.

A new science, futurology, has come into being. Conferences and symposia on futurology as well as books and reports have become part of the current scene. The approach of the year 2000 makes this science even more meaningful since besides marking the end of a millennium, what will happen in 2000 may concern many of us, and will certainly affect our students and the world in which they will practice medicine. The deliberations of the "American Academy's Commission on the Year 2000" demonstrate the extraordinary complexities inherent in any attempt to define the future. While contemporary scientific knowledge provides a basis upon which to forecast the future of technology, the future progress of science is almost unpredictable. Had we known more about the science of tomorrow, we probably would have it today.

Medical education is a sociocultural complex of values and interrelationships, and only partially a scientific discipline. When the authors ask themselves what is desirable in our age of change and choice, they are trying to foresee the future in terms of existing values. Thus, while becoming futurologists, they are not foresaking history.

Forecasting, unlike planning, does not seek actively to influence the future, and it takes into account the entire spectrum of possible options, both objective and subjective. Intuition, vision, and extravagant ideas must not be ruled out since, in the past, they have sparked off genuine "breakthroughs."

Moreover, when dealing with medical education which is mission-oriented, due consideration must be given to the human and social implications of the scientific and technological revolution. And finally, one can not ignore the political elements and processes which affect every nation's way of life, nor public opinion which serves as the feedback channel for its decision-making bodies. As a result, the art of prediction in health and health education is conceptually and technically complex. The authors have succeeded in paying due attention to all of these factors and have tried to determine the direction in which change is moving and to find some consensus of opinion with regard to the assumptions upon which a model of prediction can be constructed. This consensus is presented in the Recommendations.

The authors should be praised for having allowed any member of the team to express his individual viewpoint and present his personal comments at the end of each chapter. These comments often provide that "grain of salt" which make the book still more fascinating. The major recommendations and chapters of the book can be grouped into three main sections:

Medical education and the nation's health

Viewing tomorrow's medical education as a societal endeavor to serve the nation's health needs may be considered the authors' major contribution. They fully recognize the fact that the ultimate mission of medical education is to serve the needs of society. Therefore, medical education will inevitably become more involved in providing better health care to all. This involvement will increasingly invest the academic medical center with a new responsibility—the search for new models of health care delivery—in addition to its traditional role of creating new models of molecular biology and expert clinical performance.

Academic medicine too often complains that it has not been given the opportunity to regulate, or the responsibility to direct, health delivery systems outside of its own sphere. Actually, it never tried to assume this responsibility and often turned its back on such opportunities when they presented themselves. Medical academicians have preferred to remain in the warm and comfortable microenvironment of their medical centers. The main objective of this book is to redefine the social responsibilities for medical educators of tomorrow. They are clearly told that if they continue to disregard the community's demand for better, cheaper, and more easily accessible health care and do not educate health professionals who are aware of their community role, medical education will not fulfill its objectives and will retreat into a no-man's land. The authors call upon the medical educators of tomorrow to bring health care and medical education, two systems which for too long turned in separate orbits, into a more harmonious and effective coexistence.

This new dimension of medical education is lucidly presented and thoroughly discussed in the book's first two chapters. It runs through chapters 5, 7, and 9, and is again expressed in full in chapters 10, 11, and 12 which are probably the most controversial and challenging of the entire work. After reading these chapters, one feels that if only the academic medical community could find the strength and vigor to fight for the privilege of molding medical care delivery systems in the same way that it has traditionally defended its research and teaching privileges, we might enter a new era in medical education.

It is in this connection that the authors seek new approaches by taking a realistic view of the future relationships between academia and government. Since one cannot survive without the other, both must contribute to better communication and more understanding. The concept of government as a benevolent bill-paying agency must be replaced by a new bilateral partnership. It is the academic medical community's responsibility to educate the government in the goals and objectives of medical education and health care delivery while still preserving its own academic freedom. This may well be a long process. However, in the framework of such a collaboration, the appeal to the federal government to ultimately accept major responsibility for financing medical education (chapter 12) seems justified, and the request for 25,000 graduates per year from American medical schools by 1985 (chapter 1 and recommendation 13) quite realistic.

Expansion of medical education's scope and responsibilities

Four chapters deal with the legitimate demand to extend medical school's educational responsibility beyond the traditional undergraduate level. The expansion as formulated by the authors, will encompass moves in both directions: downwards, into the premedical, collegiate level, and upwards, into graduate, postgraduate, and continuing education. More integration of the various phases is necessary. Better integration with premedical programs will allow earlier admission into medical school, thus shortening the total medical curriculum, another prevalent trend in American medical schools. The academic health center's involvement in residency training and continuing education programs has long been expected and is a rational development. The demand for full-fledged partnership (together with professional medical organizations and government) in a coordinating body of a liaison committee on medical education (chapter 12) is well taken and could hardly be denied.

The ever-growing interaction of modern medicine with other academic fields and disciplines is another facet of medical education's expansion. The authors pay due attention to the need for cultivating links with other faculties within the university setting (chapters 3 and 6). The university setting of medical schools is already well established and will remain unchallenged. It has its roots in the faculties of science, humanities (social and behavioral sciences), and recently also in engineering and the computer disciplines. The advantages for medical education are many, but one must not deny the multiple contributions which medicine can offer in exchange.

I read and reread the book in its various drafts with growing pleasure. It is a capital contribution to American medical education, and it will undoubtedly be a high point when medical educators from the world over meet in Copenhagen in September 1972 to discuss "Educating Tomorrow's Doctors" at the Fourth World Conference on Medical Education.

Basic conditions for progress in medical education

It may be of some interest to view the book also in the context of international comparative medical education. Recently, common themes and more universal values have been emerging in discussions on medical education in all countries. This, however, has not prevented the emergence of a paradoxical situation which is most perplexing to the medical man: since each of the particular shortcomings of medical education has its own characteristic etiology in each country, what is regarded as a cause of trouble in one place is considered a remedy in another. Thus, it is only natural that some of what the authors present as desirable for American medical education in the future has been widely used (and sometimes even discarded) by other countries. On the contrary, some American principles of medical education widely applied in the United States and criticized by the authors are now being introduced elsewhere. To enumerate only a few: (1) Countries which provide "free service" to all now realize that free accessibility to such services creates consequences for which society must pay without knowing what the real needs are—free accessibility still does not mean better health care; (2) Sufficient funds for medical research do not provide the solutions to all medical problems, and the gap even widens between the best which medicine could offer and what is actually available to the total population; (3) "Open admission" into medical schools, an accepted tradition in European and Latin American countries, does not increase the heterogeneity of the social structure of medical school classes. Paradoxically enough, French universities, like some of their Latin American counterparts, recently instituted selection in admission to medical schools; (4) Women constituted some 80 percent of the medical student body in the U.S.S.R. and the Eastern European countries. Their proportion is steadily decreasing. Willingness to serve in ambulatory or primary care does not depend on sex or race, but on the organization and system of medical care; (5) Early clinical exposure and training, the old French system, once rejected by the British and Americans, is now in "high fashion" in the United States, but has recently been postponed in France where broader basic science preparation has been introduced; (6) Russia has solved its shortage of health manpower by educating *feldshers* (equivalent to physicians' assistants). This was frowned upon by Western countries for half a century. Recently, the United States embarked upon a vigorous program of physician's assistant training, while Russia is limiting their proliferation. Moreover, while upgrading is more or less of an accepted pathway in the American programs (and will probably create numerous problems in the future), it is only marginally encouraged in the U.S.S.R.; (7) In the American system, there is an explosion of allied health professions (200 are mentioned in this book) and a growing tendency for them to penetrate into the academic setting, be it college or university. The Europeans are trying to remain consistent, preserving the unity of health care and centering its functions mainly around the physician and the nurse by adapting them to new polyvalent needs; (8) The Communist countries probably succeeded more than others in keeping medical education relevant to medical care needs. Probably, this is because the ministry of health in each country is directly responsible for the medical schools which are outside of the university setting; (9) Provisions for various "tracks" of medical education within the same institution is the existing prototype in the U.S.S.R. and Eastern European countries (with the recent exception of Poland). However, this works only when free transfer from one track to another is not freely permitted; (10) The system of elective periods in American medical education is a recent advantage. Yet one may foresee a danger to the system in the growing trend towards shortening the medical curriculum encouraged by the "capitation" system. Electives will probably become the first victim of such a trend.

One should not become frustrated by all of these paradoxes and many others. They were mentioned in order to demonstrate the variety and multiplicity of experimentation in medical education and the growing need for continuing reevaluation and study. Since medical education is a dynamic process dealing with living people, it can never achieve a static balance and stop. This book proves it from its preface to its last chapter and for that, all of the authors deserve the greatest recognition from medical educators in their own country and elsewhere.

Moshe Prywes, M.D.

The Hebrew University
Hadassah Medical School,
Jerusalem, July 1972

Preface

The purpose of this monograph is to bring together the thoughts of a relatively small group of medical educators and administrators regarding the future of medical education. It is unusual in that each chapter synthesizes many hours of discussion of its authors' thoughts on the subject. It has avoided the pitfalls of two extremes: (1) the monograph that is a compilation of individual essays without any other input; (2) the staff-written document incorporating only the softest common denominators of agreement.

Each chapter of this book was initiated by two to eight knowledgeable individuals in the field who met one or more times with the chapter author to develop the outline and content for a first rough draft. These first drafts formed the point of departure for discussion at the chapter authors' first conference held in August 1970 at the summer quarters of the National Academy of Sciences in Woods Hole, Massachusetts. Transcriptions of the entire discussion were then sent to each author for consideration in revising his assigned chapter as he saw fit, leaving the possibility that it might have to be rounded out by segments of edited discussion or by dissenting opinions. Three more conferences and drafts preceded the final conference for intensive review of the finished work in September 1971. The recommendations in the front of this book represent the consensus of the coauthors as to the major thrusts of the document. These overall recommendations resulted from both the written submissions by the authors as a logical conclusion of the chapters and also from the group discussions of areas not necessarily covered in the written text. The recommendations following each chapter represent the individual author's personal viewpoint. Coauthors were also given the option of appending personal comments to any chapter; these are to be found at the end of each chapter.

How and why did this arbeit come about?

In 1967 the embryonic Board of Medicine of the National Academy of Sciences proposed a voluminous and detailed report on the future of medical education. Panels consisting of national experts in each area were appointed. Some met several times and reached logical end points for their reports; others never met. Due to a series of major problems, the grand design of the overall study had to be dropped.

At this point, a great deal of time and effort had been expended in considering the continuum of medical education. One panel had a consensus report on the future of graduate medical education and the discussions of others could be crystallized easily into reports. Except for these preliminary efforts, representatives of academic medicine had not come forth with a thoughtful blueprint for the future of medical education. This vacuum was accentuated by the publication of collateral reports such as the Millis Commission Report (1), the Coggeshall Report (2), the AAMC Conference on the "Role of the University in Graduate Medical Education" (3), the AMA–AAMC discussions on the establishment of a Commission on Medical Education, and the Carnegie Commission *Report On Higher Education and the Nation's Health* (4). The situation was discussed with Mr. Quigg Newton, President of the Commonwealth Fund, who agreed to support a more modest effort to develop a report on "The Future of Medical Education." This is the result.

Speaking for all the authors, I would like to express our profound thanks to Mrs. Judy Graves for her untiring editorial efforts in molding the various manuscripts and drafts into a cohesive final product.

William G. Anlyan

References

1. *The Graduate Education of Physicians.* The Report of the Citizens Commission on Graduate Medical Education, John S. Millis, Chairman. Chicago: American Medical Association, 1966.

2. Coggeshall, L. T., *Planning for Medical Progress Through Education.* Washington, D.C.: Association of American Medical Colleges, 1965, pp. 1–107.

3. "The Role of the University in Graduate Medical Education." Cheves McC. Smythe, Thomas D. Kinney, and Mary H. Littlemeyer, eds. *J. Med. Educ.* 44 (No. 9): 1–179, 1969.

4. *Higher Education and the Nation's Health.* A Special Report and Recommendations by the Carnegie Commission on Higher Education. New York: McGraw-Hill Book Company, 1970.

Introduction

As a result of the profound economic, social, and scientific changes that have taken place in American society over the past three decades, Americans have high and rising expectations for more and better health care. All agree that there is a great shortage of health manpower and that the need for increased numbers of physicians is pressing. The university medical school is charged with the ultimate central responsibility of educating more doctors and allied health personnel in such a manner that they will be effective in the practice of medicine in tomorrow's world.

The time for change is upon us; with education for the practice of medicine consuming a decade and a half from college through graduate training and military service, innovations to be felt by society in 1985 must begin today.

The ultimate mission of medical education is to serve the needs of society. In order to produce health manpower for the future, it is useful to know what the practice of medicine will be like in 1985. It is for such a delivery system that the continuum of medical education must be tailored. By analogy, it would be foolish to build supersonic jets while training commercial pilots to fly propellor aircraft. Martin Cherkasky in chapter 1, "Medical Education and Practice—Circa 1985," discusses the health delivery system of the future.

Chapter 2, by Lloyd Elam, emphasizes the need to seek new resources for medical and health manpower. Minority groups and women must have free access to the educational continuum of medicine with upward mobility options.

Because of the broad and special capabilities available within the university, Irving London in chapter 3 presents the great advantage of the university setting for collegiate programs in biology, medicine, and other interrelated scientific disciplines. A program in human biology such as that at Harvard–M.I.T. may contain the elements necessary for successful integration of health and medicine at the university level of education.

The problems of admission into the medical continuum are discussed by William Bradford in chapter 4, which emphasizes the bottleneck created by the lack of openings in and money for undergraduate medical education. Emphasis is made on advanced placement, premedical advising, and the problems which the students encounter in financing their medical education.

Because admission, advancement, and curriculum are closely interwoven, Gerald Austen and Thomas Kinney discuss in chapter 5 the responsibility for curriculum that medical faculties must assume if they are to process the manpower for more than two hundred health careers. These authors consider the thrust of current curricular reform from the perspective of further evolution in the future of basic and clinical sciences in undergraduate medical education.

In chapter 6, William Van der Kloot underlines the vital importance of the production of biomedical scientists to the continued advancement of new biomedical knowledge, as well as the education of the biomedical innovators and teachers for the future. Recognizing that the United States has achieved a position of world leadership in the science of medicine, Dr. Van der Kloot suggests the educational systems necessary to produce the next generation of biomedical scientists.

William Anlyan's chapter 7 embraces the area of graduate medical education as it dovetails on the one side of the continuum with undergraduate medical education and on the other with a lifetime of continuing medical education. It describes multiple careers in medicine as they relate to the delivery system.

In chapter 8, John Beck deals with the relatively unploughed yet extremely important field of continuing education. If indeed the turnover of medical information is at the rate of 50 percent every five years, continuing education looms as a vital area of concern for academic medicine.

In chapter 9, Donald Medearis and Thomas Kinney discuss the concept of a continuum of medical education extending from secondary school through postgraduate education. They highlight the need for more effective communication between medical school and undergraduate science faculty to bring about a greater degree of integration of premedical and medical curricula.

Chapter 10, "Family Practice," proved to be the most controversial and challenging chapter in the book. It was acknowledged that no book related to the future of medical education would be complete without a discussion devoted to the future of family practice. An early draft of this chapter by Dr. Stead was presented to a group of six practicing family physicians from North Carolina and Virginia. These reviewers, including an internist and a pediatrician, came to Durham in March 1971 to express their thoughts and opinions regarding the first draft and family practice in general. The productivity of the meeting led to further revision. At the August 1971 meeting of the authors, it was evident that whereas there was agreement with regard to Dr. Stead's depiction of the problems and needs, there existed a strong opposite view among the other authors as to the proposed solutions. Hence the chapter was divided into two sections, with the second synthesizing the other authors' views on Dr. Stead's proposed solutions.

Thus, the reader will recognize the difficulty and the spectrum of opinions regarding this important need of society.

Eugene Stead describes the concept and origin of the now widely accepted physician's assistant program in chapter 11. This pool of manpower, working under the physician's direction, extends the doctor's capacity for service at the community level. Such a new health career also represents a potential way-station for upward mobility in the health care profession.

In chapter 12 Ray Brown presents the very complex subject of the future financing of medical education. Unlike the relatively simple economics of single industries, medical education and its financing are an integral part of a multidimensional moiety of the economics of the health industry.

It was not the intent of the authors that this publication be regarded as the voice of any all-inclusive group or organization. The views expressed may, in some instances, not concur with those of the majority of medical educators. They represent definite positions on policy matters of importance to the future of medical education, positions whose rough edges have been (we hope) smoothed by group discussions and yet not diluted by seeking universal acceptibility.

To whom is this monograph directed? To the "deciders" who will be making decisions regarding medical education and the delivery of health care of the future. The list of deciders would include university officers, academic health educators, faculties of medicine, leaders of medical practice, members of the legislative and executive branches of the federal and state governments concerned with health care and education, foundation executives supporting innovations in health education and health care, industrial leaders whether they are directly or indirectly involved with the health care system, the consumer, and finally, of equal importance, the potential student who must ask the question, "Do I wish to enter the continuum of medical education?"

W. G. Anlyan

The future of medical education

1. Medical education and practice—circa 1985

Martin Cherkasky, M.D.

These are the days that mark another watershed in medicine. As doctors, teachers, and administrators, we are faced with ever higher-pitched demands from the general public, abuse from the despairing poor, dissatisfaction from our students, and pressing examination from all quarters of our stewardship of medical institutions.

This turmoil in the society as a whole, which has so thoroughly penetrated the university, clearly illustrates that the medical school is not the self-determining, isolated institution it has thought itself to be. The winds of change are howling down our corridors, and rather than react reluctantly and perhaps hostilely to their force, we must forthrightly examine our condition in order to understand what we must do to meet the future.

Dr. Edward D. Churchill has said, "It is important that as much as possible be learned about the hospital, because the future of this institution will be determined by society, not by the medical profession" (1). This advice, of course, applies as much to the medical school as it does to the hospital, and requires of us a hard look at values and activities within medicine which yesterday no one would have dared question. The discontent and often total disenchantment of consumers with the medical care system are mirrored vividly in criticisms of medical education by our students. They ask probing questions about the relevance of the curriculum to the practice of clinical medicine, protesting not only that there is too much basic science but also that it is taught in an uncoordinated fashion, without departmental integration. They object to the separation of basic sciences from clinical sciences and to the arbitrary division into preclinical and clinical years.

Students reject the traditional order of medical school priorities—teaching, research, patient care—and demand that they be reversed. They clamor for a say in curriculum design, threaten to boycott exams they consider purposeless, and agitate for minority groups admissions. They take up the cause of lay control and actively fight the university on behalf of community participation.

Medical education for what?

Since the purpose of this joint effort is to suggest a new design for medical education, we must raise the question: medical education for what? Before planning curriculum and subject matter for students who will be practicing doctors in 1985 and well into the next century, we must be willing to do a certain amount of crystal-ball gazing into conditions and attitudes that are expected to prevail in that society. In realistic appraisals of what medical education has been doing up to now, academicians are beginning to realize that, consciously or unconsciously, they have opted for a curriculum that is more right for them than for the students it teaches and the society they are supposed to serve.

Crucial to decisions about education of physicians for tomorrow must be estimates of the nature and extent of health care that the society will demand and support in the mid-1980s. We must calculate how health care and medical practice will be structured, the nature of the organization or framework within which doctors will work, what new types of allied health professionals must be trained and for what tasks, and what the relationship of doctors to other health professionals will be.

We must consider how ambulatory and institutional care will be related and how medical care will be financed. Will there be national health insurance? Will care be delivered primarily on a fee-for-service basis or will there be a group practice? Will there be regionalization of medical services?

We must try to foresee the degree to which the medical establishment will be willing to alter itself in the direction of communal involvement and what "community control" will mean. We must try to anticipate what new kinds of participatory relationships will evolve between providers and consumers, and how much more responsive and externally-oriented medical schools and hospitals will really become.

These are the implicit considerations that must now become explicit as we try to decide how best to prepare physicians for medical practice tomorrow. Any changes made in the curriculum will in themselves strongly influence the manner of health care delivery. By addressing ourselves to what the practice of medicine is likely to be in 1985 and devising a curriculum to make it possible, we can spur medicine to move ahead of the times instead of behind them.

The education and preparation of those who render that social service known as the practice of medicine has not been accomplished by the simple inculcation of a fixed set of professional information and skills. Rather, it has consisted of selections from an unbelievably wide spectrum of knowledge, information, and techniques relevant to the diagnosis and treatment of disease. More and more as time goes on, it must also include information of a nonmedical nature that the physician must have to fulfill the expectations assigned to him by the social, economic, and health aspirations of the society.

The nature of the challenge

Until recently, the shape, structure, form, priorities, or direction of health care did not really concern the medical student when he became a practicing physician. The health care system, its objectives, organization and operation, were naturally consistent with the expectations and aspirations of that class of society from which most physicians came—the rather narrow, middle-class and upper middle-class, white establishment. Until recently, medical care, health, life, and survival were not deemed to be the inalienable right of every American citizen. Whatever this medical elite was moved by charitable impulses to do for the rest of the society was received by these "unentitled" individuals with the gratitude one usually expresses for unexpected kindness.

What we are seeing now is clearly revolutionary. Alan Pifer, in his paper for the Eightieth Annual Meeting of the Association of American Medical Colleges said, "No longer does the special mystique of the professions render them unassailable. No longer is their authority entirely secure. The day when the voice of the consumer will be heard is here, and it constitutes a kind of revolution in our society."

It is obvious that what was acceptable twenty-five years ago is under irresistible challenge today, the very challenge that gave rise to the Millis report (2), the report of the Carnegie Commission on Higher Education (3), and now gives rise to this report. If there were not a fundamental alienation between the society we are supposed to serve and the medical establishment, it is certain that no government would have been able to slash away support for medical research, as the Nixon administration has, with the tacit acceptance if not concurrence of the population.

Science and intellectualism are now under the most incredible attack by students and the rest of society because, in their view, progress in technology has been bought at the price of human suffering and life. In the exclusive pursuit of the desirable objective that research represents, medical schools have virtually ignored other important objectives and, in so doing, have caused research to be seen as an antisocial activity and themselves as fostering the misuse of science.

Now the society is demanding that health care professionals, primarily physicians, share control over medical institutions with laymen and accept participation by nonprofessionals in critical decisions on such issues as who goes to medical school, what the community's health care priorities are, what the national health goals should be, whether hospitals should be doctors' workshops or community-oriented health centers, and so on.

It is obvious that before we can talk about student selection, medical education and curriculum, and medical care practice; before we can make plans about medical schools and their educational, communal, and research responsibilities, we must first estimate what the forces of change will produce in the way of a medical care system by the eighties and nineties. Without question, one of these forces is universal health insurance, an idea whose time has come. The many detailed proposals for national health insurance programs that have been put forth by leaders in politics, labor, and medicine and the serious consideration now being given by the Congress to national health insurance legislation are reflections of the conviction, widespread in the society, that all citizens should be enfranchised for medical care (4, 5, 6). Such proposals foreshadow the enactment of laws that will guarantee health care to all and pay for the costs of services assuring the elimination of medical pauperization before the end of the 1970s.

Recent experience with Medicaid and Medicare, however, has shown that any acceptable plan for universal health insurance must be tied to a rational system for health care delivery. At the time these programs were being deliberated, many people recognized that the infusion of more money into the medical care delivery system, without fundamental reorganization of that system, would lead to minimal improvements in care and enormous escalation of costs. The sobering experience of seeing these fears substantiated is prompting the consumer and his elected representatives to insist that the system must provide care that is both comprehensive and economic; that group practice (7, 8), and prime means by which these goals can be achieved, should be encouraged; that full advantage should be taken of technological advances (9, 10) such as the computer and its enormous potential for medical diagnosis, research and record keeping; and that the services of other health professionals (11–14) should be utilized wherever possible to aid the doctor in the discharge of his duties.

What kind of manpower?

One of the critical questions facing society concerns the shortage of health care personnel, and debate rages unabated on how many physicians are needed to insure the delivery of comprehensive, high-quality care to all Americans. This is no idle numbers game. The medical educator who is preparing doctors today for practice in the United States fifteen and thirty years from now must know whether the prime practitioner will still be the physician, supported by paramedicals, or whether primary care will be given by certain nonphysicians. Depending upon these decisions, the number of physicians we must train and the role they will play will be enormously different. At all costs we must avoid the temptation to find simplistic answers to complex problems and to solve them "on the cheap."

On the one hand, there are those who say that doctors are too well trained to do most of the things they are called upon to do and that, rather than being persons with whom the patients first comes face to face, doctors should be primarily consultants to other health professionals. If we were to follow this path, we would have to radically change medical education to train doctors as consultants and groom them for their managerial roles. At the same time, we would have to make a substantial commitment to the development of a large number of paraprofessionals or medium-trained doctors (15) and the creation of both curricula and schools to insure their standards of training. This would certainly permit us to create a large cadre of health workers far more quickly than we could graduate doctors; but in my view, the quality of care would be even less assured under those circumstances than it is now.

Still others contend that we already have sufficient health manpower and that in some specialties we have more physicians than we need (16). This conclusion is rooted in the assumption that somehow we can get the doctors we already have to practice where we want them to. But in many rural areas of this country, and in most of these where poverty abounds, there is not a doctor to be found. In the pockets where nonwhites are concentrated, and these include the core of virtually every major city in the United States, there are pitifully few physicians. Even in middle-class communities where there seem to be plenty of doctors, it's often hard to find one at night, on weekends, or at any other time when illness strikes outside of established office hours.

While it may be true that by dividing the number of presently active physicians into the total population we can arrive at a satistically acceptable physician-patient ratio, nobody in this country has yet demonstrated how we can get doctors to work where they are needed instead of where they prefer to live. So, although it can be statistically argued that we have all the doctors we need, we are not able to provide care to tens of millions of Americans.

Even in a society such as the Soviet Union which can urge people quite forcefully to work where they are needed, it has not been possible to get doctors to practice in many remote areas. Although the Soviet deficiencies in this regard are nowhere nearly as severe as ours (they have 640,000 doctors for roughly 240 million people, compared to our 325,000 doctors for a population of 204.7 million), they are planning to resolve the problem of having doctors where they are needed by increasing their number to one million, roughly, one doctor for every 250 Russians.

In considering the number of doctors now available to our society for medical care, we should not forget for a moment that a sizable proportion of those licensed each year in the United States come from abroad. Until last year that figure hovered around 2,000 or 20 percent (17) but in 1970 of the 11,032 new licenses issued, nearly one-third went to physicians who were not educated in this country (18). Should the United States be a debtor nation in so critical a manpower area as that of doctors? Certainly, our national and foreign policy objectives would be served far more effectively if we were not taking doctors away from other countries but were substituting well-trained physicians for some of the things we now export to underdeveloped nations. Assuming the span of the doctor's working life to be thirty-five years, we would need to train 70,000 more doctors every thirty-five years just to maintain the present level of supply if we were to stop depending upon foreign doctors whose training, in many instances, is greatly inferior to ours, and upon chiropractors and other nonscientific healers.

As far as our national priorities are concerned, it is curious that we must have two or three times as many of some things as the Russians have, but our nation's leaders do not even seem pressed to the point of competition in the field of health. Of course, there are those who say there will never be enough doctors. By this they mean really that there will never be enough money. There is no magic formula for turning out more doctors— the prime ingredient *is* money. A society that is now spending $70 billion a year for what is frequently second-rate and sometimes totally deficient health care is surely able to spend that much and perhaps more of its collective treasure to insure first-rate medical care for all Americans.

The Carnegie Commission on Higher Education, in its extraordinarily comprehensive and thoughtful report, *Higher Education and the Nation's Health* (19)—a document that is sure to influence the course of medicine over the next two decades—recommends a 50 percent increase in medical school admissions by 1978. They would raise the number of incoming students to about 15,300 by 1976 and to about 16,400 by 1978. In the commission's view, this increase could be accommodated by shortening the overall period of medical training from eight to six years, by increasing class sizes, and by establishing nine new medical schools. The net result would be to give the society an additional 50,000 or 60,000 doctors by the early 1980s. Such an increase, in my view, is not sufficient if medical practice continues to be based upon the physician caring for the patient, as I believe it should be.

So limited a response to the need for doctors would force us now to opt for many more less qualified medical workers who would care for the patient in lieu of the doctor. For more than fifty years, the Soviets have had extensive experience with the *feldsher*—a physician's assistant who has provided this kind of first-line medical care in Russian rural areas and in urban polyclinics as well. The Soviets are, however, not convinced that the use of such median trained people is the best way to care for their citizens. As they move toward their goal of a million doctors, they plan instead to phase out feldshers as primary practitioners. The feldsher will stand less and less in lieu of the doctor, serving rather in support of him and functioning in such areas as industrial health and health education.

Increasing the number of doctors

Central to any resolution of our health care problems is a comfortable number of properly prepared physicians irrespective of other development such as the training of new paraprofessionals or innovations in computer utilization. A substantial increase in medical school graduates would make it possible for us to end our heavy reliance upon foreign-trained physicians, meet the increasing expectations for services from all segments of the society as well as the demands that will surely grow as the population grows, and provide the society with doctors to work in the many health-related areas that have enormous impact on the well-being of individuals and communities. Of major significance is the fact that with physicians in adequate supply it would be easier for the society to encourage them to go where they are needed and, in general, to establish a reasonable relationship with practicing physicians that is difficult to do when they are in critically short supply.

In my opinion, to assure a future of more and better health care, we Americans should designate the highly skilled internist and the pediatrician as primary care professionals. This would virtually guarantee care of equally high quality to everyone. Otherwise, given the inequities in our society, those with money or some special access to the system will obtain the services of the doctors, leaving the rest of the people to the ministrations of the paraprofessionals. (Most physicians, for instance, who need care for themselves or their families, utilize the services of diplomates or fellows of a specialty college who can admit patients to the leading medical centers when hospitalization is required) (20).

If the internist and the pediatrician are to be the primary care practitioners, the 50,000 increase in the number of doctors suggested by the Carnegie Commission is far from bold enough. We would need instead to double our educational capacity, providing more than 11,000 new places in medical schools by 1978, instead of the 5,600 new places called for in the Carnegie report. In so doing we would also double the Carnegie Commission's projected increase of new doctors from 50,000 to 100,000, giving the country a total of over 400,000 physicians by the early 1980s. If we then can continue to increase medical school admissions with an additional 1,000 students each year, by 1985 we will be producing 25,000 new physicians annually, or just about double the number graduated each year in the mid-1970s.

Our experience in educating doctors during the emergency of World War II indicates that we could accomplish this end without a myraid of new schools although we would probably wish to create some in those geographical locations where there is almost a total vacuum in the medical care system. However, the bulk of the increased enrollment could be absorbed by the existing medical schools through expansion of the six-year college-medical school combination and above all by more effective utilization of all medical school facilities and faculties. This will require that academicians take a hard look at their practices and priorities and recognize and accept the fact that the *prime* responsibility of the medical school is the production of physicians to meet the health care needs of the society.

Broadening the student base

Certainly, there is no dearth of qualified candidates. The number of applicants seeking admission already exceeds, by far, the number of available spaces (21, 22). According to the Public Health Service publication, *How Medical Students Finance Their Education* (23), one-fifth of medical students in 1967 came from families comprising only 2 percent of the population, those whose yearly income was $25,000 or more. The majority, 63 percent, came from families whose income was more than $10,000 a year. Together they account for the middle-class characteristics of our medical practice. Monetary considerations have limited entry into the medical profession largely to those whose parents could pay or to those whose energies and drives were sufficient to carry them through an incredible seven or eight years of working at odd jobs while studying and serving an internship and residency. As a result, we have denied to the society and the medical profession the stimulation and enrichment that diversity could provide.

If all tuition and a modest living allowance were made available to those young people who are found to be qualified to enter medical school, if minority admissions could be substantially increased and the discrimination against women eliminated, we would be able to accomplish several important objectives. We could redress the racial and sexual imbalance, increase the number of skilled professionals imbued with a compassionate commitment to the needs of the poor, and open a new route out of the culture of poverty for many young minority people. We could also radically change the socioeconomic composition of our health care institutions.

Since statistics indicate that more than half of the doctors choose to remain in the states where they receive their residency training, medical schools drawing on local populations and providing residency training as well as undergraduate education could keep many of their new, young doctors at home (24). Therefore it would seem that the needs of the rural areas could be met most readily by establishing medical schools and teaching hospitals in the major cities that dominate these regions.

Without question, doctors will continue to flock to the suburban and urban communities which offer the most professional and personal satisfactions, leaving the ghettos and rural areas denuded of physicians. Certainly for the short term, we will have to devise means and methods for providing health care to poverty areas. One suitable mechanism, for instance, is the National Service Health Corps (25) that permits doctors to substitute service in an area of medical need for military duty. And physicians, by virtue of their knowledge and respected position in the society, must lead in a massive effort to eliminate poverty, malnutrition, and the other social ills that obstruct the health of the people. However, we cannot now devise comprehensive plans to provide medical care for the ghettos of 1985, because even to contemplate that they will still be in existence at that time is to anticipate a social failure of such profound dimensions as to nullify all our fond dreams of progress.

Designing a delivery system

As we increase the numbers of doctors available, we must, of course, design a system of medical care delivery to insure that physicians' services can be obtained with maximum benefit and economy. There is ample documentation that group practice, based upon the internist and the pediatrician as family physicians, works beautifully, achieving patient satisfaction and yielding a high quality of care with economy. The Montefiore Hospital Medical Group, for instance, met the primary health care needs of 30,000 patients with 24 full-time internists and pediatricians.

Group practice is a model with which the country has already had considerable favorable experience, and for this area of our projection we need not invent new kinds of arrangements. While local circumstances may dictate modifications, group practice will ideally be based at a hospital or closely related to it, with two-way movement of patients and staff. Services will be prepaid, internists and pediatricians will serve as primary physicians, and all necessary equipment and personnel will be available to assure diagnostic and therapeutic capability appropriate to ambulatory care. On-line medical audit will secure the quality of care, provision for continuing education plus rewards for growing skills will spur physicians to keep abreast of scientific advances, and full use of paraprofessionals will relieve doctors, not of responsibilities but of tasks best done by others. Medical students and other health professionals will receive part of their training in this ambulatory care setting, but the costs of their education will not be included in the cost of care as is presently the case as far as hospital house-staff is concerned.

Actually, we need only to examine, refine and replicate the models, such as Kaiser-Permanente (26), with which we are already familiar. In the last analysis, the success of any program is based upon its acceptance by the society. There was clear evidence of this acceptability when the Montefiore Hospital Medical Group, recently and reluctantly, terminated a prepayment plan whose capitation was insufficient to support the quality of medicine being provided, resulting in a staggering deficit that the hospital could not sustain. In this instance, 50 percent of the patients involved changed their insurance carrier so as to remain with or return to the group, even though this care cost them three or four times as much as before.

The outline of medical practice

Indications are that by 1985, the independent physician operating on a piecework basis within a cottage industry will be phasing out in urban areas. Instead of working on a fee-for-service basis, doctors will be salaried and will practice increasingly in hospital-based groups or hospital-related neighborhood health centers in locations convenient for patients. Care will be prepaid and will be available twenty-four hours a day, seven days a week. The emphasis will be on ambulatory comprehensive care delivered by the internist, pediatrician, and other specialists working in teams with physicians' assistants, nurses, and other supporting paraprofessionals. The hospital will provide backup in scientific expertise and equipment, in-patient facilities for the acutely ill, central services such as laboratory, laundry, and purchasing, as well as integrated data processing and record keeping (27). Government regionalization of health care facilities will end expensive and needless duplication of medical programs and equipment. The hospital, more closely knit than ever to the medical school, will be deeply involved in the clinical education of larger groups of medical students and graduates and also of physicians' assistants, family health workers (28), and other supporting health professionals.

With group practice arrangements universally applied, we can look for hospitalization to be reduced by about 20 percent. This one saving will have an infinitely greater effect on hospital costs than all the remedies now aimed directly at the hospital without regard for the fact that fee-for-service solo practice, almost by design, produces unnecessary hospital utilization (29, 30). Hospital costs will continue to rise with labor costs and with technological advances in procedures and equipment. However, if we reduce hospitalization through prepaid group practice and at the same time create large numbers of home care programs and nursing homes, hospital beds can be reserved for the acutely ill and patients who have passed the biological crisis will be quickly moved to facilities for less intensive and hence less costly care (31).

Quality control—an essential ingredient

It is essential that at the earliest possible time we incorporate into the health care system at all points the technique that is essential to an industrialized society, namely, quality control. The quality of care has two fundamental factors. One, patient satisfaction, merely requires that the patient make a judgment. Since the patient has no way to judge the technical quality of the services he receives, his reactions are based merely on aspects of his personal relationship with the physician and he is often satisfied with care that is abysmally poor by professional standards.

The second factor is assurance that the medical profession will protect the patient wherever his own judgment leaves him vulnerable. To this end, we must install quality control measures in the health care system that will continually monitor the quality of services the patient receives at every level and particularly in the areas of private office care and hospital ambulatory care where there are presently no audits.

Valuable indications of the quality and extent of ambulatory care could be obtained by examination of medical records to determine adequacy of the patient's medical history, thoroughness of the general physical examination, inclusion of routine x-ray and laboratory tests and the nature of follow-up procedures (32, 33). Certainly, we will need to invest some of our research resources in the development of improved and innovative techniques for quality control in health care that will provide us not only with mechanisms for assessing the correctness of diagnosis and treatment but also enable us to quantify the effects of coordination, supervision and other aspects of management on the quality of health care and the delivery system.

In 1985, in this very different medical care delivery structure manned by adequate numbers of physicians, aided and supported by paraprofessionals of many kinds working in attractive health centers and superbly equipped hospitals, fully supported by automated systems and computers, will the doctor be the same as he is today? We should hope not. While we are rearranging everything else and bringing it nearer to our ideal, we must certainly look to the education of the doctor so that he too is ready for 1985.

The coming revolution in medical education

With greater freedom to accept into medicine, without regard to economic or racial considerations, those most qualified to serve, we can choose candidates whose personal qualities and motivation as well as their intellectual capabilities indicate they will be the willing servants of society that physicians really must be. When we consider what doctors do well and what they do poorly, it is clear, for instance, that they do not understand or credit the effects of cultural and social factors upon the medical problems of individuals and the community. That is because these considerations were never implicit, much less explicit, during their training.

We will have to reorient radically the focus of medical education so that it is directed toward people and groups of people. When the basic sciences are taught primarily in relationship to the patient, the community, and the environment, doctors will readily recognize cultural, economic, and other social factors as the very warp of the fabric within which people live, get sick, get well, and die. When the doctor and his other health colleagues are taught in this way, they will not question the inclusion of the social sciences and the humanities in the medical curriculum because they will know why they must understand the anatomy of the society as well as the anatomy of the body.

The entire basic science teaching in medicine is in need of major, not minor, examination, and revision. In many instances, teaching and curriculum control are in the hands of those for whom the biochemistry, or the anatomy, or the physiology is the end point of their own academic and professional goals. It is one thing to teach biochemistry to those who will be biochemists but quite another to teach biochemistry to those who will be physicians. This is not to deny the need for basic preparation in the sciences. In medical school, however, the basic sciences should be taught in such a way and within such settings as are appropriate to the student with patient care on his mind and as his goal.

As Dr. Henry Miller, Vice-Chancellor, University of Newcastle upon Tyne comments,

> I am not alone amongst medical educators in voicing grave doubts about the continued viability of the isolated preclinical phase of medical education. For the average medical student it is a tedious and distracting chore, a penance to be undertaken before starting on his life's work. Much of what is taught is soon forgotten simply because it is irrelevant. Accurate observation can be learned in a clinical as well as in a laboratory situation, and in such a situation it has the great advantage that its importance is immediately evident. We learn easily only knowledge that has some importance for us, and we retain only knowledge we use. [34]

Within many schools there is currently great ferment and talk about care, curriculum, and integrated programs. While these point in the right direction, it is imperative for us to face up to the fact that a tenured faculty with vested interests represents an enormous obstacle not only to changes in curricula but also to all the efforts necessary to rechannel the thrust of medicine and medical education. To quote again from Dr. Miller:

> Any dean of medicine who has tried to rationalize medical education, and to evolve a genuinely integrated curriculum bridging the iatrogenic gap between its preclinical phase of biological science and its clinical stage in which scientific knowledge is applied for the benefit of the patient, knows that the main obstacle to progress in this direction lies in the powerful vested interests of the preclinical teachers.

The physician as communal healer

One of the evils that present medical education helps to perpetuate is the widespread practice of teaching medical students, interns, and residents in the degrading environment of municipal and county institutions. Here every human and compassionate aspect of care and concern for the sick is mocked by the depersonalization, the decrepit, crowded facilities, the inadequate numbers of nurses and other staff, the lack of privacy, and so on. Daily exposure to clinical experience of this character, far from fostering compassionate concern, inevitably hardens the hearts of men and demeans and diminishes the patient, the student, and the teacher. It is not without cause that the militant poor accuse doctors of, "learning on our bodies so you can become skilled enough to care for the rich," for if we would not tolerate these conditions, they could not exist.

Since the doctor of the future will be working as a member of a health team, rather than as a solo entrepreneur, he will have to be educated differently, in a milieu that is far less homogenous and exclusive than it is today. The development of new, supportive health professions and the education of candidates for them is an area where the medical schools and their associated teaching hospitals are going to have to assume broad responsibilities. By educating doctors, nurses and other health workers together, we will insure their mutual respect and lay the groundwork for the team practice of medicine.

In designing an incremental, educational system for allied health professionals that permits the students to return to the school at any point with assurance that his acquired knowledge and skills will be credited toward his advancement to the next level of complexity, we will avoid the hoax of dead-end jobs and create a true health careers ladder (35, 36). Although not all technicians, nurses or physician assistants will want to push on to the M.D. degree, this flexible system will prove for many to be the road that did not exist before.

The medium for change

It is now widely accepted by the medical establishment that in addition to its educational responsibilities, the medical school must be deeply concerned with how medical care is delivered and whether the benefits of scientific advances are made available to all people. The medical school must also assume leadership in the design and critical evaluation of new health care programs while recognizing and accepting the legitimate desire of consumers to share equally in the decision-making process.

Logically, the instrument through which the new responsibilities of the medical school can best be mediated is the department of community health. However, if a school believes that by creating even a superb department of community health it can, with only minor modifications, continue status quo operation, then the department of community health will fail and the eagerly anticipated community involvement of the medical school will not be forthcoming.

If so commissioned, the department of community health can lead the school toward effective concern for the health of groups of people by utilizing the skills of the social scientist, the epidemiologist, the ecologist, the urbanologist, the political scientist, the public administrator, and any other specialist whose expert knowledge can be brought to bear on the social and environmental origins of disease. The department of community health can help the faculty expand the curriculum to include the social sciences, sociology, cultural anthropology, and economics as well as techno-logical organizational development and the dynamics of team creation (37), thereby making medical education more relevant to the goals of the school, the students and the society.

The department of community health can also be the channel through which the medical school embarks upon the process of learning to accept consumers as equal partners in policy decisions concerning medical care and medical education, the operation of institutions and the design of programs. Community participation is not new; it's always been there, but historically, the provider and consumer have been part of the same com-munity or aspired to it. What is new is that the middle class, beset by infla-tion and the destruction of the virtues, values, and goals to which this slice of America has historically subscribed, plus the thirty to forty million poor who want a piece of the action, are beginning to clamor for the system that is responsive to *them*.

We must accept not only the fact that the wishes of society are not to be denied, but more importantly, realize that even in the most selfish sense, medicine should not try to deny them. Although the process of sharing critical decisions with nonprofessionals is basically disturbing, sometimes discomforting, and often exasperating, the process of responding to the needs of the society can activate some of the most wholesome motivations that impel men toward the profession of medicine. Our sense of fulfillment will be deeper when we have achieved a kind of symbiotic relationship between medicine and the society, a relationship that will provide for ever growing mutual confidence and respect, affection and support.

While creative departments of community health will lead in the de-velopment of effective working relationships with the community, in the design of new and rational mechanisms for health care delivery and in appropriate renovation of the curriculum and teaching goals, the real test of purpose will only be passed when departments of medicine, pediatrics, obstetrics and gynecology and all other compartmentalized structures within the school, join in an integrated attack on the problems.

If the day comes when the department of medicine itself senses its mission to be the development of community health schemes, ambulatory service programs, and health maintenance organizations and uses these programs for student and resident training, if an awakened department of medicine brings to this clinical and community medicine the same measure of commitment and scholarship that has enabled clinical science to flourish for a generation, then the role of the department of community health will change and diminish. By then the epidemiologist, the biostatistician, and the social scientist will be at home in medicine, pediatrics, and other clinical departments. If these developments materialize, the department of community health will gradually become the administrative framework within which the clinical departments will contribute their skills and will begin to turn its attention toward such management problems as hospital and group practice administration to insure that the health structures will mesh with the new capabilities.

The medical school must accomplish this major reorientation without abandoning its dedication to basic research, for it is quite clear that in the long run the way to better health lies in ever greater understanding of disease and disease processes and the development of new preventions and cures for the ills, both physical and mental, which plague mankind. Despite the current wave of anti-intellectualism, which tends to blame technology and new knowledge for the condition of man, it is man himself in his social organizations who has misused, or not used properly, the products of research.

It is, of course, true that over the past twenty or twenty-five years, a huge research establishment nurtured by generous support from the National Institutes of Health has been created within the medical schools. While this concentration on research has produced some brilliant achievements, it has also had deleterious side effects of equal magnitude. Medical education has become a by-product of scientific research, while clinical care, communal responsibility, clinical skills, patient orientation, and even, in many instances, teaching have been viewed as secondary virtues. Throughout four years of training in some of the best medical schools, the students who planned to become practicing physicians and who made up 90 to 95 percent of the enrollment, were the targets of signals, verbal and nonverbal, which said, "If you really were the very best you would devote yourself to research and teaching and not to clinical care."

Now it is time for Flexner's magnificent contribution which brought the underpinnings of science to medicine to be seen in a realistic twentieth-century perspective as equal but not superior in importance to the assumption of responsibilities in clinical communal care. We must move to join these two aspects of medical education into true partnership.

Most deans and many educators agree with this, but unfortunately much of the power in the medical school today rests with the tenured faculty who made their way not on the basis of their clinical skills, nor their communal commitments, and not even because of their excellence as teachers, but on their research papers. Tenure, which was meant to protect the academician so that he could be a radical scholar, is now the means by which the professors can adhere to the status quo and to each other, becoming an immovable mass opposing radical change. No matter how dedicated and talented those few with vision may be, they may not be able to prevail against the concentrated will of their colleagues. Deans may propose; faculty can dispose.

If indeed the medical schools are so fixed and sclerotic that they cannot take the leadership in a situation that calls for radical change, it may be that other social institutions in which the conflicts between self-serving and societal interests are not so severe will have to assume a major role in educating physicians to meet the needs of the people. For all of their enormous commitment to the academic way and to scientific medicine, the teaching hospitals in this country have, at the same time, always been pulled by their daily experience to patient care, and some even to community care. They, along with those medical schools which can shake themselves loose from the past, may, in the last analysis, prove to be the means by which the process of radical change in medicine and medical education can begin.

Conclusion

Widespread discontent throughout the society with the quality, cost, and availability of medical care and dissatisfaction with all the institutions involved in the medical care system have generated social, political, and economic forces that will mandate significant changes in medical care organization, financing and delivery by the mid-1980s.

By 1985 not only will every American be covered by a national health insurance program, but a regionalized system of group practice, hospitals, and other related resources will guarantee health care for all. This will be accomplished by a major restructuring of the financial support of the health care system involving a combination of public and private funding arranged in such a way as to reward those professional attitudes and skills, organizational developments, and cooperative relationships between all segments of the health care system without which good health care cannot possibly be made available to all.

Medical education, while based on science, will be fundamentally oriented toward clinical care. Admission criteria will be altered to select into medical school those who have qualities of humanity and personal and communal commitment as well as the necessary intellectual capabilities and an educational background that encompasses both the social and the biological sciences. The availability of funds to cover tuition and provide a modest living allowance will give those now excluded—the poor and the minorities—access to the medical profession. Together with the elimination of discrimination against women and other arbitrary forms of exclusion these changes in student admissions will produce doctors much more representative of the society as a whole.

Although hospitals will be the core from which services will emanate, the major emphasis will be on extramural and ambulatory services, with solo, fee-for-service practice being largely phased out and such devices as hospital-related group practice units, neighborhood health centers, and health maintenance organizations (38, 39) acting as vehicles of quality care. While the physician will continue to be the primary performer in the system, his practice will be enormously changed as many kinds of new health care workers, trained to assume significant responsibilities, become members of the health care team. Scientific and technological advances and continued development of computer techniques will also have wide-ranging effects, improving the capabilities and quality of care, making centralization of supporting activities possible, and bringing even those who are remote because of geography or social reasons within the protection of the system.

Self-aggrandizing competition between hospitals which results in widely uneven levels of care, costly duplication of services, and waste of scarce personnel and resources will be eliminated by local, state, and federal regulation of construction and by substitution of communal goals for narrow institutional goals (40). Any number of schematics have been developed to illustrate what relationships between medical schools, major hospitals, community hospitals, and other care resources in such a system might be (41, 42). Each envisions the medical school and the teaching hospital closely allied—with the latter having such satellites as community hospitals, health maintenance organizations or group practice units, neighborhood health centers, nursing homes, custodial institutions, and mental hospitals as well as home care and other special programs and resources that are integral parts of the health care delivery system.

We hope that well before the 1980s there will be that essential partnership between thoughtful citizens and responsive professionals necessary to insure not only the delivery of the best possible health care available at that time to all the people, but also unstinting support of research in the pursuit of new knowledge. To control and direct funding of program development, research, and education toward these ends, there must be teeth in the planning.

If by the 1980s, the selection, education, and training of the doctor, the methods of financing medical education and medical care, and the system of medical care delivery are so radically changed that the societal capabilities of medicine are equal to its scientific excellence, then, indeed medicine will be consonant with the needs of this great nation verging on the twenty-first century.

Summary

For all the virtues of some of the current legislation designed to resolve the inadequacies of the health care system in this country none goes to the point of guaranteeing health care for every American. In the next ten years federal law will guarantee health care to every American and application of quality controls will insure that this care is of the same high level for all people. Not only will a national health act cover payment of services, it will also, by incentives and other pressures, encourage regionalization of hospital responsibilities and move medical practice in the direction of hospital-related group units communally located for the maximum convenience of patients. By doubling our educational capacity and providing more than 11,000 new places in medical schools by 1978, we will add 100,000 new doctors to the pool of physician manpower, giving the country a total of more than 400,000 doctors in the early 1980s. Continuing to increase medical school admissions with an additional 1,000 students each year, we will, by 1985, be producing 25,000 new physicians annually. Shortened and innovative curricula, maximum utilization of existing facilities and faculties, and the addition of less than a dozen new medical schools will enable us to reach this goal. Federal support of medical education will make it possible for us to accommodate this increased enrollment as well as to train a large cadre of paraprofessionals to relieve the physician of tasks best done by others. The availability of modest subsidies will attract to the medical school candidates from a wide spectrum of the population rectifying the present ethnic, racial, and sexual imbalance in the medical profession. While the doctor will continue to receive a sound backgrounding in science, changes in the curricula will give him fundamental orientation toward patient and communal care. Doctors thus educated to view their health care responsibilities in broad terms will lead in the efforts to eliminate poverty, malnutrition, and the other social ills that obstruct the health of the people. Community participation in the decision-making process will be required by the national health legislation and will insure that medical education and practice are consonant with the needs and desires of the society.

Author's recommendations

1. Health care must be guaranteed for everyone and fully financed by the federal government.

2. Continuing to increase medical school admissions with an additional 1,000 students each year, we will, by 1985, be producing 25,000 new physicians annually.

3. Regionalization of health, hospital services, and hospital-related group practices should be developed and located for patient convenience.

4. Ethnic, racial, and sex-related imbalance should be rectified with appropriate subsidy programs.

5. Consumers should participate as equal partners in all policy levels in medical care and medical education.

6. New health professionals and new professional roles should develop, but the temptation to solve the problems "on the cheap" should be avoided.

7. There must be a single system and a single high standard of health care for all with rigorous quality control of all points in the health care system.

8. Health professionals should participate in a major thrust to eliminate poverty, malnutrition, and the other social ills which obstruct the health of the people.

Coauthors' comments

Dr. Anlyan:

By 1985 solo practice should be extinct. Only the very rare physician who is unwilling to work in a group situation will function as a "loner." The minimum critical mass for a "group" is three physicians, covering each other for nights off, continuing education, vacations, and most especially, day-by-day peer consultation and review. In contrast, the "loner" in solo practice has to cope with a 168 hour on-call week the whole year around except when he can arrange for a locum tenens. His time off and opportunities for continuing education are sporadic, unprotected, and if planned, usually violated by overwhelming practice responsibilities. After ten to fifteen years, the "soloist" enters the maelstrom: he is falling behind in the latest advances; he is seeing too many patients and can afford little time with each; his family life has disintegrated, and so it goes. In summary, every opportunity should be exploited in the education of the physician to acquaint him with the advantages of working with a group.

Dr. Elam:

There should not be two (or more) types of health care for if there are, the poor, the black, and the other minorities will not have equal access to high quality health care, but will be relegated to the second level of health care. For this reason, all physicians should be well trained, and no one posing as a physician (by whatever name) should have the ultimate responsiblity for patient care.

Dr. Medearis:

Expectation and reality. One of the major difficulties besetting medical education, medical research, and medical care at the present time derives from the fact that society has come to expect an almost unobtainable degree of success from technology and research. This in part must be due to the almost unbelievable accomplishments of the atomic and space ages. As medical educators, we have a responsibility to reconcile the expectations of society and the probabilities and realities of achieving an alleviation of the deficiencies in medical care with the discrepancies between what is hoped for with what can be reasonably expected and what can be reasonably accomplished. The anger directed at medical science and medical education and manifested by anti-intellectualism is in part the result of a great discrepancy between what society hopes for and expects and what can be reasonably obtained. This is not to say that great accomplishments cannot be obtained through the process of constructively addressing ourselves to the problems of medical care and human disease. It does mean that we must embark upon a very much more energetic and productive educational program through which a larger proportion of our society becomes fully acquainted with the process of medical research, its productivity, its limitations, and the relationship between productivity, effort and cost. This thesis has been eloquently developed by Dr. Donald Price, Director of the Kennedy Center for Government, Harvard University, in an article in *Technology*,* a publication of Massachusetts Institute of Technology.

Dr. Stead:

I am not convinced that all medical practice is best done by groups. In my experience, group practice is a good arrangement for handling complex medical problems and for continuing the education of doctors. The more time the doctor has for thinking, the more expensive the medical care. There are many problems of health maintenance and primary care which can be handled effectively by patterned responses which do not require rethinking of each problem. A well-integrated solo practitioner with a

---

* D. K. Price, "Science at a Policy Crossroads," *Technology Review* 73 (No. 6): 31–37, 1971.

good office staff can handle a large volume of problems more efficiently and more cheaply than any of the clinics I have seen.

The problem of solo practice is the lack of support for vacations, sickness and education. The appearance of the physician's assistant on the scene has put much more flexibility into the solo practitioner's day. The development of consortiums of solo practitioners and the doctors in medical centers to which they refer patients is worth careful exploration. If adequate support systems could be devised, the advantages of solo or duo practice would not be lost.

I am also less impressed with the benefits of putting all doctors on a salary and reducing the fee-for-service aspect of medicine. Some patients need more medical attention than the doctor believes they need. He gives this service willingly for a fee. He gives it grudgingly if he is on a salary. The patient isn't always wrong.

Dr. Wilburt Davison commented many years ago on the distribution of senior faculty giving care to patients in the Duke Medical Center after 5.00 P.M. on week days and on Saturday afternoons and Sunday. He found that the salaried doctors were not in the patient care areas but the fee-for-service doctors were. A recent check by me shows that Dr. Davison was a good observer. The distribution in the patient-care areas of the Duke Medical Center of doctors on salary and those on fee-for-service on Saturday afternoons is similar to that observed twenty-five years ago.

References

1. *The Hospital in Contemporary Life,* N. W. Faxon, Ed. Cambridge, Mass.: Harvard University Press, 1949, p. 62.
2. *The Graduate Education of Physicians.* Report of the Citizens Commission on Graduate Medical Education, J. S. Millis, Chairman. Chicago: American Medical Association, 1966.
3. *Higher Education and the Nation's Health.* A Special Report and Recommendations by the Carnegie Commission on Higher Education. New York: McGraw-Hill Book Company, 1970.
4. "National Health Insurance: The Next Attack on Medical Costs," *Changing Times, The Kiplinger Magazine,* Jan. 1971, pp. 41–44.
5. Introduction of the Health Security Act, S.4297, 91st Congress, Second Session, Aug. 27, 1970.
6. Kindig, D. A., and Sidel, V. W., "Impact of National Health Insurance Plans on the Consumer," *National Health Insurance.* Homewood, Ill.: Richard D. Irwin, Inc., 1971, pp. 15–61.
7. *Message From the President of the United States Relative to Building a National Health Strategy,* Section A: Reorganizing the Delivery of Service. Washington, D.C.: U.S. Government Printing Office, 1971, pp. 1–19.
8. *Report of the National Advisory Commission on Health Manpower.* Washington, D.C.: U.S. Government Printing Office, 1967, pp. 72–73.

9. Garfield, S. R., "Multiphasic Health Testing and Medical Care As a Right," *New England Journal of Medicine* 283, No. 20 (Nov. 1970).
10. Garfield, S. R., "The Delivery of Medical Care." *Scientific American* 222, No. 4 (April 1970).
11. Stead, E. A., "Assistants at Duke." *American Journal of Nursing* 67, No. 7: 1442–43.
12. Smith, R. A., "Medex." *JAMA* 211, No. 11 (Mar. 16, 1970): 1843–45.
13. Silver, H., "The Pediatric Nurse Practitioner at Colorado," *American Journal of Nursing* 67, No. 7: 1443–44.
14. Powell, R. N., "A Breakthrough in Medicine," *Hospital Tribune,* Sept. 21, 1970.
15. Eugene A. Stead's chapter on family practice (pp. 143–59) in this book.
16. McNerney, W. J., "Why Does Medical Care Cost So Much?" *New England Journal of Medicine* 282, No. 26 (June 25, 1970).
17. "Medical Licensure Statistics for 1969." *JAMA* 212, No. 11 (June 15, 1970).
18. "Medical Licensure Statistics for 1970." *JAMA* 216, No. 11 (June 14, 1971).
19. *Higher Education and the Nation's Health.*
20. Maloney, Milton, M.D., "The Characteristics of Hospitals and Physicians Used For Medical Care by New Jersey Physicians and Their Families, 1955–1958." Unpublished manuscript.
21. Potthoff, E. F., "The Future Supply of Medical Students." *J. Med. Educ.,* 35, No. 3 (Mar. 1960).
22. Altman, K., "Medical School Applications Up Despite Lag in Funds and Space." *New York Times,* Feb. 21, 1971, p. 1.
23. *How Medical Students Finance Their Education.* Washington, D.C.: U.S. Government Printing Office, P.H.S. pamphlet No. 1336–1, 1965.
24. *Higher Education and the Nation's Health.*
25. Public Law 623. S.4106, approved Dec. 31, 1970, establishing a National Service Health Corps.
26. *Report of the National Advisory Commission on Health Manpower,* pp. 197–228.
27. Cherkasky, Martin, "Resources Needed to Meet Effectively Expected Demands for Service." *Bulletin of the New York Academy of Medicine* 42, No. 12, (Dec. 1966): 1089–1098.
28. Wise, H. B., et al., "The Family Health Worker." *American Journal of Public Health* 58, No. 10 (Oct. 1968).
29. Trussell, Ray E., M.D., M.P.H., "The Quantity, Quality and Costs of Medical and Hospital Care Secured by a Sample of Teamster Families in the New York Area." Unpublished manuscript. July 1962.
30. Falk, I.S., M.D., "Special Study on the Medical Care Program for Steel Workers and Their Families." Unpublished manuscript. Sept. 1960.
31. *Health is a Community Affair.* Report of the National Commission on Community Health Services. Cambridge, Mass.: Harvard University Press, 1967, pp. 115–117.
32. Morehead, M. A., "Evaluating Quality of Medical Care in the Neighborhood Health Center Program of the Office of Economic Opportunity." *Medical Care* 8, No. 2 (Mar.–Apr. 1970).
33. Morehead, Mildred A., M.D., M.P.H., et al., "Comparisons Between OEO Neighborhood Health Centers and Other Health Care Providers of Ratings of the Quality of Health Care." Unpublished manuscript, presented at Medical Care Association, American Public Health Association, Houston, Texas, 1970.
34. Miller, H., "Medical Education and Medical Research" [The John Snow Memorial Lecture of the Association of Anesthetists of Great Britain and Ireland, delivered at the Royal College of Surgeons, London, on Nov. 26, 1970]. *Lancet,* Jan. 2, 1971.
35. *New Members of the Physician's Health Team: Physician Assistants.* Report of

the Ad Hoc Panel on New Members of the Physician's Health Team of the Board on Medicine, National Academy of Sciences, May 1970.

36. Levin, T., "Social Policy and Guild Policy in Health Manpower," *Bulletin of the New York Academy of Medicine,* 2nd Ser., 46, No. 12 (Dec. 1970): 1112–1119.

37. Beckhard, R., *Organization Development: Strategies and Models.* Reading, Mass.: Addison-Wesley Publishing Co., Inc., 1969.

38. *Message From the President,* pp. 1–19.

39. *Report of the National Advisory Commission on Health Manpower.*

40. *Health Planning* (a monthly publication of the Organizational Task Force for Comprehensive Health Planning), Jan. 1971, July 1971.

41. *Report to the President by the National Advisory Commission on Health Facilities,* Washington, D.C.: U.S. Government Printing Office, Dec. 1968, p. 11.

42. See Cherkasky, "Resources Needed to Meet Effectively Expected Demands for Service."

2. New resources for medical and health manpower

Lloyd C. Elam, M.D.

The major constraint to the provision of adequate health care to every-one in the United States is the lack of sufficient manpower. This is not the only constraint. Inadequate facilities, lack of funding for some segments of the population—particularly the working poor—inefficient delivery system, and failure of consumer acceptance in some areas are all impediments to adequate health maintenance. None of these obstacles can be overcome, however, unless there are great increases in manpower. If the nation becomes committed in the next few years to the notion that every-one is entitled to health care of high quality and that it is in the best interest of the country to provide it, will there be an adequate number of trainable persons to supply the necessary manpower? The policy of health care as a right has been widely articulated in the past decade. At the same time, many do not believe it is possible to train enough manpower to give high quality care.

It is now estimated by some that we need 100,000 additional physicians, and that without the 1,500 doctors from other countries who are licensed yearly, we could not keep our medical centers going at their present rate. Whether or not this is true, it cannot be doubted that we have a critical shortage in certain localities. The medical schools produced 8,240 new doctors in 1969, which was an increase from 6,502 in 1950. As medical schools continue to expand their classes to provide additional doctors, the question of the source of the students must be raised. Is it broad enough to effect a change in the maldistribution of physicians? The actual size of the existing pool of individuals interested in studying medicine is un-known. We do know that only one-half of those who apply for medical school are admitted, and also that fully half of those rejected prove them-selves able to master medicine by going to foreign medical schools or entering American schools later on. To provide continuing growth of medical schools along with socially desirable heterogeneity of the students, it will be necessary to turn to largely untapped sources of applicants. This chapter will be addressed to the necessity of finding new manpower sources for medicine and utilizing these resources in ways that will insure adequate distribution and efficient use.

Existing sources of medical manpower

Medical students in the past have come from a small segment of the population. Admission requirements have forced most of them to pursue a similar biological science curriculum in college. They have generally entered medical school directly after college and have thus been in their early twenties with little work experience outside the academic setting. Their fathers have been in the middle- and upper-middle-income brackets and, more often than not, were themselves sons of professionals.

Relatively few of the nation's colleges have provided most of the medical students. Bartlett points out that "in 1954, 162 institutions provided 75 percent of the entering class of the nation's medical schools, while the entire number of colleges represented in all medical schools was 708. Similar figures for 1964 are almost identical, 75 percent of entrants from 156 colleges with the total representing 741 colleges and universities" (1). With a total of 1,239 colleges and universities in the United States, this means that no medical students came from 498 educational institutions.

The number who come from minority groups is disproportionately small. In the years prior to 1969, approximately 2 percent of the medical class was black, three-fourths of these being in the two predominantly Negro medical schools—Meharry Medical College and Howard University. Figures for other minority groups in the 1968 first-year classes were: American Indians, 3; Mexican Americans, 20; and Puerto Ricans, 87. (Nine percent of the students were women) (2).

The geographical origin of students shows the largest proportion coming from the Middle Atlantic states and the smallest number coming from the East and South Central states. This may, of course, be related to financial patterns between different geographic areas.

One other aspect of traditional sources of medical manpower relates to the motivation of the student. Students who come from professional families have a tendency to make career decisions early and, being aware of the difficulty of getting into medical school, structure their college careers to assure admittance. One of the most important motivational factors has been the availability of enough money to pursue a medical career. Many more students than the number who apply are motivated toward medicine when they enter undergraduate school; financial considerations are among the most potent dissuaders. Not only must the student have funds to support an expensive education, he must also forego an income for a very long time.

The result of these and other factors (such as the criteria for choosing students) has been until recently an extremely homogenous medical student body along a number of parameters. This gives some advantages to the educator, but the resulting disadvantages for delivery of health care have initiated a trend toward a more heterogeneous student body.

The need for new manpower resources

The existing sources of medical manpower have not been exhausted. Even if medical schools greatly increased their intake of students to correspond with the larger number of students attending undergraduate college, their classes could still be filled by traditional methods of selection. There has been very little change in the percentage of baccalaureates who go on to medical school. Actually, there has been a slight decrease in the percentage of persons earning baccalaureate degrees who then go into medicine. In 1960, 3.9 percent of persons earning baccalaureate degrees entered medical school. By 1970, the proportion had dropped to 2.9 percent (3). This drop was entirely due to the increased number of young people without a corresponding increase in the number of places in medical schools. Not only are there two applicants for each opening; there are also many more students who would apply if there were more places. Why then do we need new sources of students for biology and medicine?

One of the main reasons that health care is poor in the United States is the uneven distribution of providers. For example, in the black ghetto, the ratio of physicians to population is only 1 to 5,000 and in many rural areas it is worse. This compares with 1 to 640 in the general population. Because there is evidence suggesting that doctors coming from rural and ghetto surroundings are more likely than others to practice there, ways must be found to recruit more students from these areas of great need. Eighty percent of the graduates of Meharry Medical College, for example, practice in the rural and urban ghetto.

In addition, the development of new systems of health care can be enhanced by drawing on sources that would yield a larger percentage of persons interested in team or group practice. Doctors already work long hours, and if they are to provide more services, they can do so only by having more helpers. The traditional medical student, who is seen as a highly competitive, very individualistic person—one who prefers doing things himself instead of delegating—must be supplemented by students who can function with division of labor. There will be a growing reliance by the population on groups, teams, and corporations for medical care. The success of these newer modes will depend in large measure on available manpower who will prefer them to individual practice.

Perhaps less obvious as a reason for developing new manpower resources is the need to give all persons with ability a chance to enter the health professions. The great underrepresentation among black, American Indian, Spanish-speaking, and other minority groups will not be solved simply by increasing the number of places in the medical school. If there is truly to be equal opportunity, ways must be found to fill some of the new places with minority students. The rewards to society for giving the minority student an equal opportunity to become a physician will be better health care and with it an improved economy in his community. Not only is adequate health care a stimulus to employment of paramedicals and supportive personnel, but it is a major factor in attracting industry into a community.

Recent efforts to increase the number of black physicians

The amount of effort which has recently been expended on increasing the number of black physicians is remarkable, and has produced information that can serve as a basis for further development of these and other resources.

Negroes for Medicine by Lee Cogan, a report of a conference sponsored by the Macy Foundation and National Medical Fellowships, summarizes efforts to increase the number of blacks in medicine and in college through 1967. Support of continued education for exceptional students and grants to institutions to improve their instruction in science constituted the major programs. It is difficult to assess their effectiveness in increasing the number of medical students because of the very limited opportunities for Negroes to study medicine. However inadequate their number, these grants (from Rockefeller Foundation, Rosenwald Fund, and National Medical Fellowships) resulted in a stable number of Negroes entering medicine and in an improvement in the quality of their education. The conferees saw the necessity for an ongoing program of active recruitment.

In 1954, when the Supreme Court outlawed racial segregation in the schools, two medical schools (Howard University School of Medicine and Meharry Medical College) were educating more than three-fourths of the Negro physicians. These two schools had more applicants than they could admit, and it was obvious that many black applicants were being denied admission because of lack of space. The first hope was that integration would solve the problem. The expectation was that since the doors of many schools were now open, black students would enter all medical schools in proportion to their representation in the population. For a few years, some foundations made grants and scholarships available to black students if they would attend a predominantly white medical school. Despite these approaches—eradication of racial discrimination in admission policies by many schools and subsidies to black students for attending white schools—there was an actual decrease in the total number of black students enrolled between 1955 and 1964.

From 1965 to 1971, activities in many areas were aimed at increasing the number of black medical students. Among the most important was the change in policy of the medical schools from passive acceptance (or rejection) of black students to one of active recruitment. Primarily, medical schools had done practically no active recruiting, since there was always an abundance of applicants. The pressures responsible for this change came from medical students, medical faculty, the federal government, the association of medical colleges, the black community, and other sources.

Many schools welcomed the challenge and appointed recruitment committees made up of faculty, students or a combination of both. It was soon discovered that recruitment of blacks was more effective when done by blacks. Many of the principles which apply to athletic or other kinds of recruitment applied here. Personal contact, early acceptance, flexibility—all became part of the recruitment program. In a few schools, it was felt that the presence of a black person high in the hierarchy would provide a role model, would show that the intent of the institution was genuine, and would give the school an official who could take primary responsibility for publicizing its changed image regarding blacks.

Coupled with these efforts was a marked increase in financial aid. It is estimated that 90 percent of black medical students must receive financial assistance because they come from families with incomes below $8,000. A milestone in medical education was reached when federal loans and grants became available to needy students through the medical schools. For the first time, many schools were able to admit students who did not have money. The number of black applicants began to increase.

Some institutions gave inducement grants to attract the best students. There is insufficient evidence to draw conclusions about their value either in increasing the number of blacks in medicine or in widening the arena from which they are obtained. These grants may have merely shifted the top students from one institution to another. After more experience, we will know if they were given to students who would not otherwise have gone to medical school.

Other organizations worked with the medical schools to increase the number of black students during this period of 1965–1970. Foundations such as Commonwealth, Kellogg, and Maurice Falk Medical Fund were among the first to give support to the black medical schools for both strengthening their programs and expanding. The Sloan Foundation led the way in grants and fellowships to black students to go to the schools of their choice. The Macy Foundation and later the Carnegie Foundation were the most active in increasing the awareness of the need. These foundations and several others supported recruitment and enrichment programs in a large number of medical schools and undergraduate colleges. The federal government, through the Health Professions Improvement Act, made it possible for the predominantly black and the predominantly white medical schools to modernize, increase the size of faculties and student bodies, and develop flexibility in curriculum. This created the environment for recruitment of a more heterogeneous student body.

Once the pattern was established, other governmental agencies and non-governmental organizations became aware of ways in which they could support the effort. A further step was the reconsideration of admission procedures, but this activity has not gained uniform acceptance. Specifically, some schools set up minority admissions committees and because of the fact that the Medical College Admission Test was less predictive of ability in black Southern students than in others, they placed less emphasis on the scores in this test. In one school, students were admitted in a special category so they could make up academic deficiencies while they studied medicine.

Increased recruiting activity has been successful. The number of Negroes applying to all medical schools and being accepted has increased at a faster rate than the rate of increase for whites. It is not possible at this point to give a formula for successful recruitment, but a comparison of the more successful and the less successful programs seem to indicate the following essentials:

1. Money to subsidize 90 percent of the black students recruited. This alone is not sufficient to recruit a student but is the most important single factor.

2. Reasonable assurance for the student that if he begins, he is likely to graduate. This need is not peculiar to these particular students, but may be a factor when the number of minority students is extremely small.

3. Multiple facets consisting of short-range active recruiting techniques and longer-range activities to increase the pool of well qualified persons.

Problems encountered in increasing the number of minority students

Three major problems have been encountered repeatedly with the above activity. The most important is the size of the applicant pool. Unless the pool of applicants is expanded, efforts to increase the number of minority students may result in a few applicants going to the highest bidder. If the acceptance of minority students begins to approach 100 percent of those applying, the danger exists that adequate selection criteria are not being used. Although the traditional selection criteria are not being applied to these students, some criteria must be developed to predict which are likely to become the type of doctor needed by society.

Another problem relates to the minority student who is admitted on a noncompetitive basis. Should there be special programs for him? Should he have tutors and flexibility in his curriculum? Should he be guided in special directions, encouraged to specialize in certain fields? Does this student have special adjustment problems and should arrangements be made to help him solve them?

A third problem relates to the reaction of the nonminority student who must compete for admission to medical school and if unsuccessful, feels he has been displaced by a noncompetitive minority student.

These three problems cannot be ignored. The pool of minority applicants must be increased, we simply cannot continue to increase acceptances from the existing small pool of applicants. Increasing the size of the pool will solve the problems of noncompetitive admissions because there will be an adequate pool of competitive minority students. Meanwhile, there must be programs to meet the individual needs of the minority students. As the medical school develops special programs to meet individual needs, it will find that all students need a similar curriculum, one which takes into consideration their strengths, weaknesses, and in addition, their special interests. As to the third problem the total number of new places in existing and new schools exceeds the number of minority students being admitted but the problem will not be completely alleviated until the opportunity to study medicine is open to every student with adequate ability and the desire to practice in areas of need.

Mechanism for tapping new manpower resources for the future

Using the experience gained from recent efforts to recruit blacks into medicine, we can now project a fairly comprehensive approach to the expansion of manpower resources for medicine generally. No comment will be specifically made about other health professions, but the same general principles will probably apply. No specification is made for the type of health care system which should exist, but the assumption is that it must be one that distributes providers equitably into every segment of the population.

Ethnic minorities

Ethnic minorities provide the largest under-utilized potential source of medical manpower. The mechanisms for remedying this situation must be multiple, because the causes have been multiple. Among the causes have been prejudice on the part of medical school admission committees, the cost to the student, low expectation by students regarding the possibility of admission, lack of role models to stimulate interest in young students, lack of good counselling, inadequate preparation for a variety of reasons, and lack of a long-range program for continued increase of the ethnic minorities in medicine.

Active recruitment by medical schools can go far to convince students that the medical profession does need additional manpower from minority, as well as other, sources. Techniques of recruitment will vary in different situations and will include: (1) the use of minority representatives as recruiters; (2) recruiting through the mass media; (3) advertising; (4) encouraging interest of minority group institutions, educational and non-educational, in getting more students into medicine; (5) competing with industry on special occasions, such as high school career days, plus a variety of other methods.

It is not enough to be interested in more students from ethnic minorities. It is likewise not enough to have programs to meet their individual needs. Even if such programs are established and coupled with active recruitment methods, the effort may remain unsuccessful because of coexisting needs for manpower in other areas that do not require the long nonearning periods essential to medicine. Increased efforts to recruit ethnic minorities for medicine will stimulate competition from other fields for these same students. Therefore, the total pool of ethnic minority students for graduate and professional education must be increased if we are to do more than shift a group of students from one area of graduate study to another. In order to do this, three courses of action are recommended to colleges: (1) Make counselling available to guide the student in the direction of his greatest ability and interest instead of allowing him to base his decision primarily on monetary considerations; (2) Develop cooperative programs, electronically assisted teaching, and stronger science courses to prevent students from developing weaknesses in paramedical areas; (3) Collaborate with a medical school in the teaching of premedical courses; this will also help the medical school update its curriculum.

In trying to reclaim some of the potential applicants who have not had these advantages, medical schools can offer a supplementary course in the summer, post-baccalaureate courses and a flexible curriculum to allow special work during the first two years of medical school. In launching such special programs, it is important to emphasize that this additional effort on behalf of minority students is justified because of the unique contribution they will be able to make, so that faculty and legislators, among others, do not take patronizing, hostile, or otherwise defeating attitudes toward these students.

It is recommended also that some undergraduate schools should become health science schools and with programs directed toward developing graduates for medical studies. Students in such a college would be able to major only in health-related fields. If a small predominantly Negro college agreed to do this (for example, a college in the Atlanta University consortium), it could put all its resources into a common area and provide a kind of excellence not possible under the present system. If a community college which existed in a predominantly Mexican-American community should do this, it would speak clearly to the residents in the community of its relevance to that community.

Those whose families are poor

Society has revised its policy concerning who deserves medical care. In the past, it was consistent. Only those who could afford it received care and only those who could afford it were educated to provide the care. The educational restraints now far outweigh the service restraints and the disequilibrium helps create an unnecessary disproportion between supply and demand for services and of manpower to supply the services. The assumption has been made, or so it seems, that if a family is poor, its children do not have as much ability as the rest of the population—except for the rare child whose outstanding ability forces recognition despite the obstacles. Fortunately, this assumption is being discarded.

The cost of a medical education is prohibitively burdensome to the poor family. If students are educated in a system where the economic hardship is unjustly harsh, are they likely to be concerned about economical ways of doing things when they are on the receiving end? Medical education should be free from beginning to end. For example, if the student goes to an undergraduate health science school, if he enters a special program of health career studies, or if he enters the system at the medical school level, he should not have to pay tuition. At higher levels, stipends should approximate the real cost to the student. The number of students who could become physicians through this method would make medical care for the poor feasible. A quick calculation will show that the expanded earning power thus created would bring about complete repayment of educational cost to the federal government in the form of income tax. For example, in 1968 the average annual income of post-baccalaureate males was

$12,938 (4) and the average net income of general practitioners was $32,308 (5)—a difference of $19,370. The income tax on the difference with standard deductions would easily amount to $4,000 and over a forty-year career would bring the government $160,000.

Women in medicine

The United States is notably deficient as compared with European countries in tapping the sizeable pool of women who might go into medicine. Only South Vietnam, Madagascar, and Spain have fewer women in medicine, proportionately, than does the United States. Seventy-five percent of the physicians in Russia are women, but in 1970, less than 10 percent of the places in United States medical schools went to women (6).

Why are so few women in the "Land of the Free" going into medicine? Dr. Catherine McFarland, research professor of gynecology at Woman's Medical College, now the Medical College of Pennsylvania, has suggested that "college vocational counselors are the single most potent force steering women away from medicine," although there are doubtless other forces, equally as powerful but not so readily identifiable, which take place as a part of the acculturation process. Dr. McFarland points out that counselors exaggerate the difficulties of getting a medical education and promulgate false fears of professional handicaps for women.

One might expect to find the admissions committee of the all or largely male medical college the next stumbling block to women pursuing a career in medicine, but a check of the number of male and female applicants against acceptances by United States medical schools from 1930 to 1960 shows that the percentage of applying women accepted is practically the same as the percentage of men. The problem lies in the fact that so few women apply. In 1962, 13,251 males and only 1,166 women applied for admission to medical school in the United States (7).

One factor that does mitigate against women in the admissions committee's considerations is their higher attrition rate. About 8 percent of the male students drop out, but more than 15 percent of the females drop out, most of those for "nonacademic" reasons. Those women who continue are found to perform at least as well as men; and in 1970, about 20 percent of the women graduates were in the top 10 percent of their classes (8). Receiving an M.D., however, is not the end of the struggle for the women in medicine; further obstacles lie in their path. Many medical educators and clinicians have strongly advocated that women be directed into "suitable" medical specialties. Psychiatry, pediatrics, obstetrics and gynecology head this list. Proscribed for women are surgery, endocrinology and orthopedics (9). In addition, there is the generally held attitude that specialty training for a woman may be a "waste" of time and funds, because she may drop out of practice to raise a family or may work only part-time.

The United States is in a period in which national and personal values are being reassessed. In all likelihood, the definition of "wasted time and effort" will be subjected to repeated scrutiny, and especially so, since physicians are in such short supply. No doubt women will be expected to continue to devote their time to the early years of child rearing, but the demand for physicians will enable them to work part-time if they desire and there will be less talk of wasted effort referring to effort spent educating women for medicine.

Some schools are beginning to make allowances for the sometimes erratic schedules of women in medicine. Woman's Medical College makes provisions for maternity leave and a staggered curriculum (10).

Some medical schools have considered setting up nurseries for infant and preschool children. Such magnanimity is not without its beneficial effect, but other action, more to the point, must be taken within United States medical centers. Courses must be given which point up male-female role falsification and distortions in our society, not only so that more women may be recruited into medicine but also to resolve some of the psychological problems resulting from distorted role definitions. Efforts must be made to enlighten students, clinicians, and administrators about their female colleagues and "fellow" students. They must realize the extra burden they themselves often assign these students in the form of their traditional expectations of women.

Some educators may be enthusiastic about recruiting more women for medical careers but exclude the Negro female, since she is seen as a matriarch. She too suffers from stereotypy, and must be considered as a potential medical school applicant.

Although medical schools can and must make an effort to recruit and retain women in the profession, society in general must shift its traditional expectations. There are indications that this shift has begun, and that medical schools can add to the momentum and benefit from it by articulating their policy vis-a-vis women applicants.

Sources of medical manpower other than colleges

The present development of physicians' assistants includes four main categories: (1) Nurse-practitioner and nurse-specialist practitioner; (2) Former corpsman retrained as doctor's assistant; (3) Nurse midwife; (4) Pharmacist. There seems to be little doubt about the ability of such individuals to enhance the delivery of health services. The pattern of use varies. In some instances, the physician's assistant works in very close contact with the doctor, performing many duties which he would otherwise perform but leaving definitive care to the doctor. In other cases, he works quite apart from the doctor, performing definitive procedures but always with a physician available in case of need. The physician's assistant will undoubtedly develop many skills and increasing knowledge with experience. Some will eventually want to study medicine to become physicians themselves. Although these will probably be few, they will likely be an important group for they will often have practiced in rural areas, where physician's assistants and nurse midwives are most welcome, and might therefore want to return to these areas as practicing physicians. Since present admission policies for medical school are based on experience in college, it would seem wise for the Association of American Medical Colleges and the American Medical Association to begin studying the situation now with a view to developing guidelines for medical schools that will certainly want to accept some of these men and women.

What has been said of the physician's assistant is to some degree true of other allied health professionals. Most of them, when they wish to become physicians, will be competing with college students under the same criteria. Some will have enough experience so that the medical school will want to accept them and give them credit for their previous work.

An easier and more obvious source of medical manpower will be the movement of cerain practitioners into a different relationship with other doctors. The osteopathic physicians, the optometrists, the podiatrists, and the pharmacists have not contributed optimally because they are not in close association with the M.D. As other changes occur in the medical care system, they will relate differently, but with only slight effect on the manpower shortage since these persons are already engaged in health care.

The future of one important group is difficult to predict. That group, the consumer advisory council, is made up of many persons with keen interest and a great deal of knowledge about medicine. They will likely become a source of manpower, but whether they will prefer managerial and allied health areas or will be a source of physician manpower cannot be forseen at this time.

Pre-college level activity to develop health career interest

It is well known that children begin to form impressions very early which will later determine their career choices. For this reason, many programs aimed at the college level reach only those persons who have leaned toward a medical career since childhood. The most effective stimulus in early childhood has always been the repeated one-to-one contact with a physician who impressed the child. The yield from programs at this age is low, however, and the time lag is so great that efforts here can only be a part of general education.

In high school, specific programs are recommended to stimulate interest in a health career. High school counselling is enhanced by a closer relationship between counsellors and a nearby medical school. Teachers of health and health related subjects would perform a great service if they had at least some of their health training in the medical center rather than having all of it from teachers unrelated to medicine. "Career day" programs and other special programs often help to kindle interests.

High school is not a good age to use coercion or enticements, because most high school students are in their early teens. They are in the early process of personal identity development, and commitment to a career at this time would deny them the moratorium which many students need to work out problems of identity. If such a moratorium is not allowed, decisions may be made that may not be suited to later developing personality characteristics. On the other hand, if courses in health sciences were supported so that they could become more "science" and less "hygiene," as is the trend in the better schools, the adolescent would incorporate the orientation to health science in his total development.

Possible results of tapping these new medical manpower sources

Many troublesome questions can be asked about the consequences of utilizing these new sources of manpower. Will over-saturation become a problem, that is, will the supply exceed the demand? What will happen to the quality of the student body? What will happen to the attractiveness of medicine as a career? Will it become difficult to attract the best students if the class becomes too heterogeneous? Will the consumer lose some of his respect for the doctor? Are government and private sources likely to continue to support medical education?

Despite these and many other unanswerable questions, the course is clear. The alternative is to prolong a health care, manpower, and cost crisis which is no longer acceptable to the American people. In the next few years, more manpower will be demanded and new sources will be found. Fertile among them will be the black, the American Indian, the Spanish-speaking American, women and the poor. Other sources as discussed in this chapter will combine with these to yield sufficient numbers to provide the medical manpower for the type of health care discussed in other chapters.

Summary

The demand for more doctors has been recognized. In the past, physicians have been selected from a narrow segment of our population and given a uniform type of education. The emerging health system will best be served by enrollment of medical students from all economic, social, and ethnic components of our society and from both sexes. This heterogeneity can be accomplished through active recruitment, as a variety of successful recruitment programs are demonstrating. The fact that the already large pool of applicants for medical school can be expanded by recruiting those who have been excluded in the past because they were black or poor or went to the "wrong" college, suggests that there are ample human resources to man an ideal health system and that it is unnecessary to turn to a system where doctors will be in short supply. The problems which are created by opening up new sources of manpower while medical schools are unable to accept all the applicants from present sources must be faced, but cannot be completely solved until there are opportunities for everyone with the ability for and interest in studying medicine. Even in the projected future when there will be many more places and perhaps open admissions, active recruitment will still be necessary to provide a heterogeneous mix of medical students.

Author's recommendations

1. Active recruitment should be used in insure that adequate numbers of applicants from all segments of society be educated as physicians and that the number of places in the medical school be determined by the number of physicians needed for health care rather than by any notion that there is a shortage of human resources.

2. Medical education should be free to the student from beginning to end, subsidized by the federal government.

Coauthors' comments

Dr. Cherkasky:

There is a great deal of discussion, concern, and even some action surrounding the need to bring into the medical profession people who have hitherto, for a variety of reasons, found themselves systematically excluded.

This includes blacks, Puerto Ricans and the poor of every racial group. Many people now view this exclusion as unfair and want to see the condition rectified with equality for all. While this, of course, is a legitimate position, it seems to me that the need for including hitherto excluded people is even more important than the desire to be fair. Medicine as a social institution has suffered because its membership has been drawn from so narrow a segment of the society. In fact, as one examines the response of organized medicine to social needs and social problems, it is clear that the goals of the upper middle-class segment of our society, from which most doctors have come, have been identical with the goals and objectives of medicine. If health care is to be the right of all the people, it is important that medicine itself be broadly representative of all the people. Otherwise, the social, cultural and other characteristics which provide diversity among Americans and make the nation unique and strong will not be reflected in medical practice, or its sensitivity to the needs of the large groups of people for whose health care it is becoming responsible. Also, significant thought must be given to the role of women in medicine. In the Soviet Union, more than 80 percent of the physicians are women and, without in any way attempting to simplify a very complex question, I want to point out that the delivery of primary ambulatory care seems to be accomplished very well by them.

Dr. Medearis:

I want to take issue with the short shrift given to the subject of women in medicine in this chapter. The present form of medicine is highly discriminatory against women. That must not be the impact of this chapter or book!

Carol Lopate's book, *Women in Medicine,** communicates well the problems of being a woman interested in or in medicine today. She recommends, and I concur, that (a) "the national climate of opinion concerning sexual roles be changed so that many more high-calibre women will, of their own choice, decide to become doctors . . . ," and (b) the double burden of being a woman and a medical student / doctor be lightened by changes in admission policy, curricula, residency training, and board requirements which do not change quality. This is possible. All these facets of the subject are thoroughly discussed and documented in her book and need not be dealt with further here. But this chapter and this book should recognize that a revolution, an orderly one, is occurring as it must and that women in medicine will have an enormous impact on medical education. That subject alone deserves the same extensive consideration that all of us

* Baltimore, The Johns Hopkins Press, 1968.

have given the content of this book—and this book is deficient to an extent—for our having failed to deal more thoughtfully with this matter.

References

1. Bartlett, James, "Changes in Entering Medical Students' Preparation for the Study of Medicine," in Robert G. Page and Mary H. Littlemeyer, eds., *Preparation for the Study of Medicine* (Chicago: University of Chicago, 1969).
2. Cadbury, William, "Program for Increased Enrollment of Minority Group Students in Medicine," unpublished manuscript written for the National Medical Fellowships, Inc.
3. Association of American Medical Colleges Committee on the Expansion of Medical Education Report, *J. Med. Educ.* 46, No. 2, (Feb. 1971): 105–116.
4. "Consumer Income." Current Population Reports, U.S. Department of Commerce Bureau of Census Series, No. 74, p. 60.
5. *Profile of Medical Practice,* Chicago: American Medical Association, 1971, p. 67.
6. Morgan, Beverly C., M.D., "Admission of Women into Medical Schools in the United States: Current Status." *Woman Physician* 26 (June 1971): 305.
7. Ibid., Table 1, p. 309.
8. Ibid., p. 308.
9. "Women's New Role in Medicine," *Medical World News,* April 10, 1964, p. 78.
10. Lee Cogan, ed., *Negroes for Medicine* (Baltimore, Johns Hopkins University Press, 1968).

3. The college and university in medical education

Irving M. London, M.D.

We live in an age of anomalies. Great intellectual and scientific achievement coexists with extensive ignorance and illiteracy, and great wealth with grinding poverty. In the past three decades the pace of progress in the biological and medical sciences has been more rapid than at any previous time in human history, and yet large segments of the world's population, even in some advanced countries, suffer from inadequate health care. Small wonder that higher education generally, and medical education specifically, reflect the incongruities and malaise of our society, and that thoughtful critics question the objectives of our educational systems.

For the past six decades, medical education in the United States has followed the recommendations of the Flexner report, namely, the establishment of university standards and performance for medical faculties and students and a four year medical school curriculum of preclinical sciences and clinical medicine. These recommendations initiated a revolution in American medical education with many salutary results. A strong base in the preclinical sciences was established as a prerequisite for clinical medicine, and the quality of clinical practice was greatly enhanced.

Like many revolutions, however, the Flexner revolution was incomplete. To establish university standards, medical schools were to be "articulated" with their universities. Since most medical schools were built near hospitals rather than on the main campuses of universities, the articulation of the medical schools with their universities was, at best, very loose. In general, the geographic separation of the medical school from its university was accompanied by the intellectual isolation of the medical faculty and students from the rest of the university. For many years, the improvements in medical education engendered by the Flexner report obscured the disadvantages that derived from such intellectual isolation. But in recent years, these disadvantages have become more obvious.

Biology and medicine are increasingly dependent on a wide range of other scientific disciplines. For the past few decades, biology has derived great benefit from chemistry, and the field of biochemistry has become central in importance to the life sciences. More recently, the biologist has been seeking a more profound and precise understanding of living matter with the aid of the mathematical, physical, and engineering sciences. The penetration of these sciences into biology and medicine has great potential and promise, equivalent in character to the impact of chemistry on progress in the biomedical sciences. Medicine, which is not only a biological science but is also a major social activity, is dependent on the social and behavioral sciences, public administration, management, and law. Indeed, one may fairly argue that the wide gap that exists between the potential of the medical sciences and the actuality of health care derives in part from the insular relationships of medical education to these other sciences and disciplines. It is very difficult, however, to bring these various disciplines to bear on biology and medicine in the setting of most medical schools. Scientists of high quality generally prefer to work as integral members of their respective departments or at least in close proximity to their peer groups.

The separation of the medical school from the university has been responsible in part for another problem, the lack of educational opportunities in human biology for students not directly involved in the study of medicine. Human anatomy, human physiology, and human pathophysiology have been the province of the medical school and have been largely inaccessible to nonmedical students. It is distressing to find that the well-educated American college graduate is very often quite ignorant of the structure and function of the human body.

Still another difficulty inherent in the separation of medical education from general university education is the discontinuity in the educational process which obtains between the years in college and the years in medical school. Too frequently, there is little coherence between the curricula in college and the curricula in medical school. Students in college and graduate school have difficulty pursuing their interests in human biology; students in medical school have difficulty continuing their studies in areas that were of major interest to them while in college, despite the fact that such studies are often directly relevant to biology and medicine.

In considering biomedical education of the future, we propose not only to recognize the difficult problems that derive from the current system of medical education, but to suggest solutions to these problems in the framework of major changes in the character and setting of education for health and medicine. Educational institutions are responsible for the production of the manpower needed for the provision of health services, for the planning, design, and operation of health care systems, and for the creation of the new knowledge essential to progress in health.

Many kinds of skilled manpower are needed: these include physicians, dentists, and public health experts; life scientists, especially those oriented toward human biology; bioengineers; health services planners, managers, and administrators; medical economists and sociologists; political scientists and lawyers concerned with the planning and operation of health programs. The education of such health professionals involves many disciplines: the clinical disciplines and their subspecialities; the public health disciplines such as nutrition, epidemiology, biostatistics, and environmental health sciences; the biomedical sciences, including the morphological sciences, biochemistry, physiology and pathophysiology, microbiology, and pharmacology; bioengineering, biophysics, biomathematics, computer science, systems analysis, and operations research; psychology, sociology and anthropology; economics and managerial sciences; political science, public policy analysis and public administration, law and ethics.

The development of educational programs for such a wide range of health professionals requires the resources of universities and cannot be achieved within the framework of medical schools alone. It might be argued that the medical schools should be concerned only with the education of physicians and that other health professionals should be educated in the various other branches of a university. The attitude reflected in this argument, however, would tend to prolong the intellectual isolation of the medical school.

We propose the development of educational programs with the following objectives: (1) to integrate education for health and medicine into general university education and to promote the spirit and values of liberal education in the education of health professionals and scientists; (2) to develop the interfaces of biology and medicine with the other natural sciences and with the social and behavioral sciences, management, public administration, and law; (3) to promote continuity and coherence in curricula that begin in college and extend through graduate or predoctoral study into the period of postdoctoral fellowship or internship and residency; (4) to promote flexibility and enhance opportunity for students to pursue highly diversified programs suited to their individual interests and talents and appropriate for the development of new or emerging health professional career paths.

A crucial element in the integration of education for health and medicine into general university education is the development of a coherent curriculum in human biology which is available not only to students of medicine but to a wide range of other students as well. An important feature of this program is the teaching of human biology as a continuum beginning at the level of the college undergraduate and extending through graduate study, whether for the M.D. or Ph.D. degree, into the postdoctoral period.

Human biology has been variously defined. Medawar suggests that it stands for a new conception of the natural history of mankind.

> Human biology is not so much a discipline as a certain attitude of mind towards the most interesting and important of animals. . . . It is about men rather than man, about their origin, evolution, and geographical deployment; about the growth of human populations and their structure in space and time; about human development and all that it entails, of change of size and shape. Human biology deals with human heredity . . . ; with human ecology and physiology, and with the devices by which men have met the challenges of enemies and of hostile environments. Human biology deals also with human behavior. . . . Finally, and most important—because most distinctively human—it must expound and explain the nature, origin, and development of communication between human beings and the non-genetical system of heredity founded upon it. [1]

Perhaps the simplest definition would be the study of the interaction of the biological and behavioral characteristics of man in his adaptation to his environment.

The study of human biology deserves a central place in university education. Human biological characteristics have a determinant influence on the social, political, economic, and cultural behavior of individuals and groups. Our society is challenged to make wise decisions on increasingly complex issues such as population planning, control of environmental quality, the allocation of resources for health needs and educational programs, and the control of drug abuse.

It should not be assumed that physicians and other health professionals are knowledgeable in the field of human evolution or human genetics, population biology, or human behavioral development. Medical education stresses the diagnosis and treatment of illness and tends to neglect seriously these important areas concerned with the biological characteristics of man. And only too often the molecular biologist, the biochemist or the microbiologist knows much too little of human biology and is unaware of the exciting scientific challenges in the study of man in health and in disease.

There are various ways in which a curriculum in human biology may be organized. New curricula are being developed at several universities including Oxford, Stanford, the University of California at LaJolla, and in the framework of the Harvard–M.I.T. Program in Health Sciences and Technology. Although the curricular organization may vary, there seems to be considerable agreement on the contents of a curriculum in human biology. At the undergraduate collegiate level, a curriculum in human biology includes general biology, human evolution, human genetics, the organismal biology of man, human behavior, and human ecology.

General biology is concerned with molecular and cellular biology and proceeds from the molecule to the organism and from the microorganism to man. It deals with the properties of living matter, the synthesis and replication of macromolecules, the molecular and cellular mechanisms of genetics, the biochemistry and biophysics of cellular metabolism, the organization of cells, tissues, organs, and organ systems, and the correlation of structure and function at these different levels of organization. In describing the natural environment in which organisms live and evolve, it introduces elements of climatology and geology.

Evolution is the essential unifying principle of the biological sciences. It is the study of the evolution of organisms and of environments, of natural selection working on genetic variation. A curriculum in human biology emphasizes primate and human evolution and as such is concerned with comparative anatomy and physiology.

Human genetics studies the principles of the origin and transmission of the biological characteristics of man. These principles can be learned from many organisms and some are best or exclusively illustrated among lower forms of life. This study deals with the interaction of heredity and environment and with the applications of genetics to human health and disease. It comprises human biochemical, behavioral, and population genetics.

The organismal biology of man is the study of the structure and function of the human body, i.e., human anatomy, physiology, and biological anthropology. It is concerned with the human body as a whole, with individuals and with groups, with human somatic variation, and with the long-term adaptation of populations to environmental stimuli.

Human behavior is viewed as man's adaptation to his environment, and human institutions are seen to evolve as adaptations based on the biological characteristics of man. The study of animal behavior, especially of primates, and the behavioral and social patterns of early man and of contemporary primitive man are included in this field. Human behavior is concerned with the biological bases of human sexuality, human aggression, and socialization. It includes behavioral genetics and the development of human behavior and personality; it seeks to understand the interface of the human brain and human behavior, and studies chemical influences on behavior and biological factors in psychiatric disorders.

Human ecology comprises the relationships of human biology, habitat and culture. The unit of study is the human population, its size, structure, dynamics and relation to its environment in respect to food, energy, and material resources. Human ecology is a meeting ground for a wide range of scientific disciplines, including demography, epidemiology, nutrition and toxicology, the environmental sciences and engineering, the social sciences and law.

The foregoing curriculum in human biology is an integral part of a continuum and may be followed by more advanced study of the structure and function of the human body in health and in illness. This more advanced curriculum includes the human morphologic sciences, anatomy and pathology, human biochemistry and physiology in normal and abnormal states, pharmacology, microbiology and immunology. It is an integral part of the education for the M.D. degree or the D.M.D. degree or for a higher degree in public health.

At the interface of human biology with the other natural sciences are biophysics, biomathematics, and bioengineering. This interface comprises a broad spectrum of studies of which some illustrative examples may be cited: control mechanisms in living systems, mathematical models of biological systems; biomaterials sciences; fluid mechanics in the human circulation; musculoskeletal mechanics and joint function; visual, auditory, and tactile psychophysics; the physiology, acoustics, and perception of speech; artificial intelligence; the applications of computer science to medical information systems and diagnosis; biomedical instrumentation and the engineering of health care systems.

The penetration of the physical sciences and engineering into biology is designed to deepen our understanding of living systems and to apply these disciplines to the solution of important health problems. Such penetration is one of the objectives of the Harvard–M.I.T. Program. A rigorous introductory course in physics has been developed with many of the illustrative examples derived from human biology and pathophysiology. Courses in human anatomy, physiology, and pathophysiology are being developed and taught jointly by human biologists and physical scientists. Research on major health problems is being undertaken in a multidisciplinary approach designed to join the physical sciences and engineering with the biological sciences in common efforts. We believe that the vigorous interaction of these disciplines in common educational, research, and health care programs will result in the productive development of the interface of human biology with the other natural sciences.

The interface of human biology with the behavioral sciences is concerned with neuropsychology and social psychology. Neuropsychology deals with the neural sciences and human behavior, with the neurobiologic basis of human behavioral development and of human mental illness. Social psychology is concerned with group behavior and with the social institutions which evolve in response to the interaction of human societies and their environment, an interaction conditioned by the biological characteristics of man.

Human biology has many interfaces with the social sciences, some of which comprise the field of social biology. This field comprehends a wide range of studies: environmental quality and environmental health; nutrition, food production, food standards and toxicology, agricultural economics, and the politics of agriculture and food production; the social effects of health and medical practice, e.g., the prolongation of the average human life span with its social, political, and economic consequences; the ethical issues involved in population control and in genetic intervention; the potential effects on the human gene pool of the survival of individuals with deleterious genes and the converse, the early recognition of genetic defects and their correction, control, or elimination; the effects of social policies and practices on human health, e.g., the effects of urbanization on population density, pollution, housing, and the availability of public services; the influence of tax policies and religious practices which may encourage or discourage population control; or the impact of compulsory health insurance on the provision of health services.

A major interface of the social sciences with human biology and medicine is that concerned with the provision of health services. This includes the economics of health care, public policy, and public administration; the politics of public agencies and of the professional associations concerned with the provision of health services; the planning and management of health services.

In proposing the development of a continuum in human biology beginning at college level, we do not intend that a college major in human biology be the sole or the preferred path to a medical education. Admission to medical school or to an M.D. program should be open to a wide range of students interested in many different majors or fields of concentration, in the humanities and social sciences as well as in the natural sciences and engineering. The availability of courses in human biology would offer such students the advantage of an educational experience that is valuable in itself, one that should also be of help as they try to decide whether to pursue a career in the health sciences or medicine. In emphasizing a curricular continuum in human biology that extends into graduate and post-doctoral study, we do not wish to minimize the value of a baccalaureate program in human biology. Such a program should qualify fully as a field of concentration appropriate for students seeking a liberal education whether or not it extends into graduate study. College undergraduates should be able to enter combined degree programs, e.g., a bachelor's degree in human biology and higher degrees in biology or in related fields; or a bachelor's degree in one of the natural, social or behavioral sciences or engineering and a higher degree in human biology, medicine, dentistry, or public health. Students should have numerous options and the programs should be highly flexible to allow changes in direction without undue loss of time.

The products of these educational programs should reflect the wide range of competences required for the provision of health services, the planning and operation of health care programs and the creation and transmission of new knowledge in health and medicine. Some examples of the products of these programs may serve to illustrate the objective we seek to achieve, namely, the progressive penetration of the natural and social sciences into biology and medicine and the development of an informed social and behavioral analysis of the human goals and costs and the human meaning of health activities. Graduates of these programs will include:

1. Physicians and dentists with a strong scientific base in engineering and the physical sciences, or in the behavioral and social sciences, e.g., a cardiologist with a knowledge of electrical engineering, an orthopedic surgeon with mechanical engineering skill, a dentist with an understanding of biomaterials science, a neurologist or psychiatrist firmly grounded in the neural and behavioral sciences, a physician-administrator with extensive knowledge of economics and public policy, public health experts with a deep appreciation of human ecology.

2. Life scientists oriented toward human biology and concerned with human evolution, genetics, nutrition, and ecology as well as with the structure and function of the human body in health and in disease.

3. Psychologists concerned with human behavioral development, normal cognitive processes, learning disabilities, and behavioral disorders.

4. Biomedical engineers engaged in the application of engineering to biological systems and to the solution of health problems, e.g., bioengineers concerned with control systems and instrumentation for life support mechanisms, biomaterials scientists involved in the development of materials required for artificial organs and prosthetic devices, experts in fluid dynamics seeking a deeper understanding of cardiac function and blood flow.

5. Health care planners, systems engineers, and managers; community designers and architects involved in the development of healthy environments and effective health-care institutions.

6. Economists, political scientists, and public administrators concerned with public policy for health and medicine.

7. Sociologists and social psychologists who can study the influence of social and cultural attitudes toward health and illness, can perceive the health needs of individuals and groups and can evaluate the social institutions which are developed to meet these needs.

8. Lawyers with the knowledge and motivation to advance the public interest by putting the law to work in behalf of the health and medical needs of our society.

The future development of education for health and medicine should engage, we believe, the resources not only of medical schools, dental schools, or schools of public health, but the resources of the universities as a whole. Medical education will prosper if it is effectively integrated into general university education. It is not our intention here to offer a detailed blueprint of a university curriculum in the health sciences. We prefer to present a general concept of an educational program in human biology and the health sciences and their interfaces with the natural, social, and behavioral sciences, and to indicate the roles which the products of such a program can play in our rapidly evolving society. We recognize that the interests, resources, and styles of universities vary greatly and that many variations on this general theme may be developed. We believe, however, that this concept provides a desirable framework and orientation for the further development of medical and health education.

Author's recommendation

Education for health and medicine should be integrated into general university education. A crucial element in such integration is the development of a curriculum in human biology which would offer a continuum beginning at the level of the college undergraduate and extending through graduate and professional study into the postdoctoral period. The curriculum would include the study of the evolution, genetics, behavior, and ecology of man, the structure and function of the human body, and human pathophysiology. At a more advanced level, it would include the study of the clinical sciences or the public health sciences or the life sciences oriented toward human biology. The interfaces of human biology with the other natural sciences and with the social and behavioral sciences should be developed through multidisciplinary educational and research efforts. These programs should be designed to produce physicians and other health professionals required for the provision of health services and for the planning and operation of health care programs, and scientists and educators needed for research and teaching in the health sciences. These objectives may be achieved by the development of close collaboration between various schools of a single university or by the establishment of interinstitutional programs linking colleges, universities, or professional schools.

References

1. Medawar, R. B., "Foreword," *Human Biology: An Introduction to Human Evolution, Variation and Growth*. Harrison, G. A., Weiner, J. S., Tanner, J. M., and Barnicot, N. S., Eds., New York: Oxford University Press, 1964.

4. Requirements for admission to medical school

William D. Bradford, M.D.*

At the present time, admission to medical school in the United States is a bottleneck through which neither the number nor the diversity of manpower needed to operate present or future systems of health care can gain entrance to the continuum. In seeking ways to open up the constricted area of medical school admissions, it is appropriate to consider: (1) the advantages and disadvantages of the present system of admission; (2) the need for a better system of selection; and (3) the possibility for multiple systems of medical school admission.

The present system

In 1971–72 there were 29,000 applicants for admission to medical school and 12,361 were enrolled, an acceptance rate of only 42.6 percent (Table 1). The simple fact is that there are not enough places in our medical schools for all qualified applicants. Such a situation creates undue competition among eligible candidates and defeats all attempts to alleviate the physician shortage. On the basis of Medical College Admission Test (MCAT) scores alone, it is estimated that 75 percent of the applicant pool may be qualified for admission to medical school (1). If this assumption is correct, more than 7,690 qualified applicants were unable to enter medical school in 1970 (2). These statistics can only suggest the frustration and unhappiness that affect the lives of several thousand young people who want to enter medicine today and will affect even more in the next few years. Estimates based on census figures indicate that applicants for ad-

* The author is solely responsible for the content of this chapter but is indebted to the following individuals who met as a group with the author for a day's discussion of medical school admissions: William G. Anlyan, M.D., Duke University; John L. Caughey, Jr., M.D., Case Western Reserve University; Thomas D. Kinney, M.D., Duke University; Irving M. London, M.D., Massachusetts Institute of Technology and Harvard Medical School; and Donald N. Medearis, Jr., M.D., University of Pittsburgh.

Table 1.   Trends related to medical school applications for first-year classes entering 1962–1973

Entering year	No. of enrollees	Individuals filing applications	Applications filed	Number of MCAT examinations *
1962–63	8,642	15,847	59,054	15,165
1963–64	8,842	17,668	70,063	17,271
1964–65	8,836	19,168	84,571	19,323
1965–66	8,760	18,703	87,111	18,966
1966–67	8,991	18,250	87,627	18,922
1967–68	9,473	18,724	93,332	19,706
1968–69	9,863	21,118	112,195	22,288
1969–70	10,422	24,465	133,822	26,562
1970–71	11,348	24,987	148,797	28,896
1971–72	12,361 †	29,000 ‡	200,000 ‡	33,869
1972–73	12,900 ‡	35,000 ‡	245,000 ‡	45,324
1973–74	13,300 ‡	35,000 ‡	245,000 ‡	46,000 ‡

* Taken during preceding year
† Based on AAMC Fall Enrollment Questionnaire
‡ Based on comparative estimates
Reprinted with permission from *1973–74 Medical School Admission Requirements, U.S.A. and Canada.* A.A.M.C., 1 Dupont Circle N.W., Washington, D.C. Chapter 3, "The Medical School Admission Process," pp. 16–29.

mission to medical school will continue to increase until 1975, when those born in the record year of 1953 will be ready to seek careers in medicine. Conservative projections of baccalaureate degrees to be awarded suggest that 28,000 candidates will apply to medical schools in this country in 1975 and that 34,000 will apply in 1980 (3). If these figures prove accurate, medical schools could be faced with 21,000 "qualified" applicants in 1975 and 25,500 by the year 1980 (2).

At the present time, medical schools do not become aware of possible candidates until they identify themselves by applying. By the time the application is received, the candidate has completed three years of collegiate work under the guidance of his premedical advisor. The competitiveness of present admissions requires that the candidate present a record of "scholastic achievement and intellectual potential." Freely translated, the chief ticket for admission to medical school is a record of high grades, especially in the sciences. The present emphasis by admission committees on science background is illustrated in Table 2. Biology, organic chemistry, and physics are almost universally required premedical subjects. Candidates are also required to take the MCAT which is designed to measure verbal and quantitative ability, general information, and science achievement. Most students who are admitted score over 500 in all categories on this

Table 2. Summary of required premedical subjects for 1973–74 entering class *

	Number of medical schools (N = 114)		Number of medical schools (N = 114)
Biological sciences:		Humanities:	
Biology (unspecified)	106	English	76
Cell biology	2	Foreign language	7
Comparative anatomy	2	Humanities (unspecified)	6
Embryology	8	Mathematics:	
General biology	7	Analytical geometry	6
Genetics	8	Calculus	18
Molecular biology	1	College algebra	10
Zoology	3	College mathematics	6
Chemistry:		Mathematics (unspecified)	19
Biochemistry	1	Trigonometry	8
Chemistry (unspecified)	69	Physics:	
General chemistry	13	General physics	57
Inorganic chemistry	28	Physics (unspecified)	49
Life science chemistry	1	Social and Behavioral Sciences:	
Organic	110	Anthropology	1
Physical chemistry	2	Behavioral science (un-specified)	10
Physical chemistry or quantitative analysis	1	Psychology	6
Qualitative analysis	17	Social science	8
Quantitative analysis	18	Sociology	3

* Figures based on data provided fall 1971.

Reprinted with permission from *1973–74 Medical School Admission Requirements, U.S.A. and Canada*, A.A.M.C., 1 Dupont Circle N.W. , Washington, D.C. Chapter 1, "Premedical Planning," pp. 1–5.

test (Table 3). College grades and MCAT scores are, then, the major academic requirements for admission.

Attempts to gauge motivation, nonintellectual talents, and extracurricular activities of candidates are sought in recommendations from their college professors. These documents, usually checklist forms, substantiate the college grades and MCAT scores and indicate desirable personal traits such as character, implying honesty, responsibility, and integrity. Recommendations are an important resource for admission committees, the more so when the writer is well known to the committee. Unfortunately, they do not always show whether or not the candidate has pursued courses for which he is most eligible, nor do they estimate the degree of difficulty of the courses taken. Recommendations and applications do not always allow an in-depth view of the student's nonacademic activities nor reveal how productive he may have been in areas such as journalism, social work, or

Table 3.   Percentile ranks for selected MCAT scores for 1970–71 first-year applicants who were accepted and for total applicants

Selected MCAT scores	Percentile ranks of MCAT subtest scores *							
	Accepted applicant group				Total applicant group			
	VA	QA	GI	Sci	VA	QA	GI	Sci
705	98	86	97	98	98	91	98	99
655	84	67	86	90	88	77	90	94
605	63	45	68	71	73	60	76	80
555	44	25	43	43	56	40	55	58
505	25	12	24	20	37	23	34	35
455	12	06	09	08	21	12	16	19
405	04	02	02	03	09	05	04	09
355	01	01	00	01	03	02	01	03

* The Medical College Admission Test (MCAT) subtests are: Verbal Ability (VA), Quantitative Ability (QA), General Information (GI), and Science (Sci). Percentile rank is the percentage of each group earning a score below the selected score.

Reprinted with permission from *1973–74 Medical School Admission Requirements, U.S.A. and Canada*, A.A.M.C., 1 Dupont Circle N.W., Washington, D.C. Chapter 3, "The Medical School Admission Process," pp. 16–29.

student government. Recent studies indicate that within the upper ranges of intelligence, assessment of how well students run "on their own power" may be more important than grades in predicting successful careers (4).

The personal interview provides for an exchange of information between applicant and admissions officer. The properly conducted interview individualizes and personalizes the selection of students and permits evaluation of the applicant who "looks good on paper." At this time, further assessments of temperament and motivation are made. The interview carries critical weight in the admissions process, and a negative comment by the interviewer frequently has the effect of a rejection.

The undergraduate origin of the medical school applicant is of importance and more than casually related to his success. The list of institutions from which the bulk of entering medical students comes has been remarkably constant over the past two decades despite increases in colleges, student enrollment, and medical schools. In 1954, three-fourths of the entering freshmen in medical school came from 162 institutions (5). One decade later, in 1964, three-fourths came from only 156 colleges (6). Michigan, Illinois, Harvard, and Columbia usually head the list of schools providing the most medical school entrants, but a group of small, highly selective liberal arts colleges makes a constant contribution as well (5, 6).

Advantages of the present system

Because medical schools are faced with a very large pool of highly qualified applicants to fill a limited number of places, it is understood that only candidates who are likely to graduate will be admitted. In reality, this has favored selection of students with strong science backgrounds and high science aptitudes because they are the most likely to survive. Furthermore, the selection from such a large pool of very capable candidates favors students with four years of college experience, and very few who have not received a bachelor's degree enter medical school. In summary, present selection methods are based on the widely held assumptions that: (1) academic grades and MCAT scores are uniformly measurable and applicable to the applicant pool and therefore, presumably fair; (2) selection based on science grades and MCAT scores has produced a low attrition rate in medical school in that 90 percent of all medical students who enroll now graduate; and (3) every physician needs an extensive background in science to practice medicine.

Disadvantages of the present system

The first assumed advantage of the present admission system, emphasizing high academic achievement in the sciences, has produced escalation of the grade point averages (GPA's) and MCAT scores required to gain admission. All medical school catalogues extol the virtues of the broad liberal arts education, but when the chips are down, only the applicants with top grades in science get in, and the students know it. The disturbing feature of this posture is that high GPA's and MCAT's are not predictors of performance in the clinic nor in the practice of medicine. If we continue to select students on the basis of higher and higher grade point averages in science and higher MCAT scores, it is likely that the pool of candidates will become increasingly limited and biased. In 1969–70, only 3.2 percent of baccalaureate degree recipients applied to medical school (3)! The selection of future physicians from such a small pool may provide too narrow a base for our health manpower and may exclude the different categories of manpower that will be essential to the health needs of society in future decades.

The second stated advantage of the present system is that its criteria of selection have produced a low attrition rate. This certainly is true, and there is nothing wrong with low attrition; it is a commendable attainment. It is well known that most medical school attrition occurs in the first two years and that fewer students drop out in the third and fourth years, so what the admissions office has actually done in selecting students with high grades in chemistry, mathematics, and physics is to guarantee successful completion of the first two basic science years of undergraduate medical education (7). This practice has, however, eliminated from medicine many students who would be strong in clinical, managerial, or social areas of the profession. We have established no guidelines to success in the clinical years, and in fact have no really clear idea of the credentials and traits that correlate with success in lifelong careers of clinical medicine.

The third stated advantage of the present system of admission is that every physician needs a strong background in natural science to practice medicine. During the past two decades, society has heavily underwritten basic research, with the result that more scientists are alive and productive today than at any time in history, and the turnover in scientific fact is tremendous. Medicine and society have surely benefited from the influence of basic science in the medical schools, for the creation of new knowledge is essential to progress. Unfortunately and unintentionally, however, this influence has heavily biased the selection of medical students. By insisting that all come to the first year with the ability to pass highly sophisticated courses in physiology, biochemistry, and microbiology, we have set too many hurdles that a prospective student must clear in order to survive in medical school. All too often, failure in one basic science course has meant failure in medical school. The bias toward science is also reflected on the collegiate scene. When a student with an otherwise strong record gets a "C" in organic chemistry, he risks being refused admission to medical school and all too often is counseled toward some other field. Medical school faculties must reconsider whether the natural science base is the only background from which our future physicians should originate. It is worth conjecturing that outstanding college students with majors in psychology, economics, business, and history might constitute a diversified and talented pool from which to select future health manpower.

Financial aid

Aside from restricted admission, another major obstacle to the study of medicine is money. A student today must either come from a wealthy family or incur heavy debt. Students are increasingly unable to finance themselves and seek financial aid. There is a wide variation in the cost of medical school education because of widely varying tuition charges, ranging from $206 per year at some state universities to more than $3,247 at many private schools (Table 4). Tuition is only part of the cost of a medical education. Food and lodgings constitute a major share of total expenses for all students. Seventy percent of all medical students live in

Table 4. Estimated minimum expenses for first-year students at U.S. medical schools, 1973–74 *

First-year expense item	Private schools			Public schools		
	range	median	average	range	median	average
Tuition and fees						
resident	$ 518–3,247	$2,500	$2,344 } †	$206–2,000	$ 850	$ 879
nonresident				$576–2,710	$1,846	$1,833
Room and board						
(minimum)	$1,000–3,000	$1,700	$1,716	$700–3,500	$1,500	$1,542
Books and supplies (not including micro- scope)	$ 175–600	$ 300	$ 302	$100–525	$ 250	$ 288

  * Data provided fall 1971 by 48 private schools and 66 public schools.
  † Seven private schools report lower tuition fees for residents than for nonresidents.
  Reprinted with permission from *1973–74 Medical School Admission Requirements, U.S.A. and Canada*, A.A.M.C., 1 Dupont Circle N.W., Washington, D.C. Chapter 4, "Financial Information for Medical Students," pp. 30–39.

apartments or houses which cost considerably more than living at home or in school-owned or controlled accomodations. The average annual expense for room and board is $3,636 for a single medical student and $5,780 for a married student without children and living in a house or apartment (8).

More than three-fourths of the annual income for all medical students in 1968 derived from three sources: (1) spouses' earnings (29 percent); (2) gifts and loans from family (25 percent); and (3) own earnings and savings (24 percent). Other sources of income, in decreasing magnitude, were gifts and loans from outside the family, nonrefundable grants (scholarships, grants in aid, tuition remission, etc.), and other sources such as G.I. Bill and military reserve pay (9). It is interesting that the spouses' earnings provide almost half the total income for married medical students with no children, while single students draw heavily on their families and their own earnings (8, 9).

Financial aid in the form of low-interest, long-term loans and scholarships is available for medical students if they prove need, and in 1969–70 approximately 41 percent received financial aid from their medical schools totalling $4 million in nonrefundable grants (10). The vast majority of medical students who request loans receive them and the average loan is $1,479. In many schools, less than $10,000 per year is available for scholarships and loans. It is likely that more demand will be placed on this source of funds as medical school tuition and inflated living costs increase.

In sharp contrast to the limited financial aid for medical students are the resources available to Ph.D. candidates in the medical sciences, for whom training grants provide stipends of more than $3,000 yearly, plus free tuition, without consideration of financial need. Federal support of Ph.D. programs has amounted to about $25 million a year in direct aid for students who number less than one-fourth the total of medical students (11). Nonrefundable grants accounted for only 3 percent of the income reported by medical students in 1967 (8, 9).

The need for a better system of admission to medical school

Changes evolving in society, the American university, and in medical education dictate that restricted admissions to medical school do not serve the best interests of the nation. Society presently has high and continually rising expectations about the scope, quality, and availability of health services, and is moving insistently toward the goal of optimal health care for all citizens (11). In the past two decades, higher education has undergone great changes (12, 13), some of which are: rising academic standards, increasing numbers of students, more diversified social backgrounds of these students, increasing specialization of faculty, increasing independent study programs and elective curricula, a change in the liberal arts concept to include in-depth study in one field by students, and the greater participation of the university in community affairs. In the medical center there are increasing academic pressures on students and faculty. The appearance of molecular biology as the major substrate of premedical, preclinical, and basic science material has led to overlapping and repetitious course material and has unduly influenced the admissions committees. There has also been increasing specialization as both students and faculty seek fulfillment of their own individual interests and needs.

In seeking a better system of admissions, one of the fundamental questions to be answered is: What role will the M.D. graduate play in future systems of health care delivery? Possible solutions to this question are discussed by Dr. Cherkasky in the first chapter of this book and by Dr. Van der Kloot and Dr. Anlyan in their respective chapters on the "Education of Biomedical Scientists" and "Graduate Medical Education." With prospective roles and goals for the future identified, it should be possible to work backward, recruiting and educating the different kinds of physician to be needed.

The present system of medical school admissions cannot be improved without responsible guidance and aid from the sources traditionally involved in medical education. These are the Association of American Medical Colleges (A.A.M.C.) at the national level, the medical schools themselves, the premedical advisors at collegiate and university levels, and others such as the family physician, specialists, and educators. The A.A.M.C. has assumed responsibility for giving premedical students information about admission requirements for medical schools (10). It might also consider an active role in career guidance by advising these young people about the many other career possibilities in biomedicine and health-related fields. Its active Group on Student Affairs might give consideration to longitudinal studies that could identify early characteristics of collegiate and medical students who later qualify to enter the critical fields of future health care delivery systems. Studies are badly needed on how to influence career selection. Admission committees should seek the help of educational psychologists in evolving selection criteria for nonintellectual and personality traits of medical student applicants. Simply stated, we need to find ways to identify the qualities in a student that will make a good doctor.

At present, there is very little hard data on individual characteristics as related to career choice. For example, in selecting students who will enter public health, what do we have to know about them and how do we have to train them? Similarly, what talents, interests, and personal traits characterize the student who will become a generalist physician, surgeon, internist, or pediatrician? Some raw data on many of these questions can be found at the Association of American Medical Colleges, in the Case Western Reserve University study on medical school graduates, in a *Survey of American Pathologists* (14), and in an ongoing Duke University study on attitudes and motivations.

A hard look must be taken at the role and responsibilities of the medical school faculty in admissions. Because of the admirable impact of basic sciences over the past two decades, heavy emphasis has been placed on credentials in hard science. This in turn has dictated the processing of premedical students through collegiate curricula. In future years, the custodians of public philosophy will likely choose to emphasize delivery of health care. To keep pace with public expectation and to man the more than 200 career slots that the proliferation of biomedical knowledge has created, medical schools must admit a much broader base of talent. Medical students should include future scientists as well as the large group who will plan and deliver patient care, head health teams, and involve themselves in the economic, legal, and public policy affairs of medicine. By assuming more responsibility for admissions and processing of physicians, the medical school faculty can widen the scope of medical education and in this way fulfill its broader obligations to society.

It is impossible to consider the problems of admissions apart from those of curriculum and promotion because they are of one cloth. At present, we are not only selecting students for curricula which fail to meet our needs, we are forcing them through a lock-step series of basic science courses within the medical school. We are saying that all medical students must prepare for and pass the same courses in biochemistry, microbiology, physiology, etc., that all must have had identical basic science experiences before they can practice medicine. A fuller realization of the increasing competence, diversity, and ability of the pool of collegiate talent should move us to provide gradations of courses in basic science to fit the needs of the individual student instead of the needs of the basic science department. As we are increasingly flexible in our clinical curricula, we need to move toward greater flexibility in basic science. In such a system, the student would be placed in the basic science cource designed for his own background and motivation. In this way, the advanced science student would respond to challenge and move ahead, and the student with a nonscience background would achieve a basic understanding. In no instance should failure in one basic science area, such as biochemistry, mean total failure in medical school.

Importance of the premedical advisor

The role and responsibilities of the premedical advisor are of paramount importance for he is the first contact many students have with the field of medicine. The premedical advisor sets the image of medicine at the undergraduate level. Very few of them, however, are physicians familiar with medical education and clinical medicine or are even remotely concerned with society's needs in health manpower. As early as 1953, it was clear that passably effective premedical advisory systems were not common and thoroughly satisfactory ones practically nonexistent (15). The stated duties of the premedical advisor are to help the student select the right courses, to counsel him in times of academic or other trouble, to supplement the efforts of classroom instructors to stimulate an appreciation of the life of the mind, and to guide the students in making future plans. For one man to discharge all these duties successfully is difficult in a small liberal arts college and impossible in a large university. With increasing numbers and specialization of both faculty and students, it is unlikely that one or several part-time advisors can take enough time and energy away from teaching and research to do a good job of premedical advising. Perhaps it is in the small liberal arts college that the role of premedical advisor is best fulfilled. Here the advisors, formerly biologists but more recently chemists, or even a group of scientists, can get to know their students both in and out of the classroom, thus forming a close student-teacher liaison. In the large university where premedical advisors are faced with hundreds of students they do not teach or know, such liaison is impossible.

With appreciation of the problems inherent in making an advisory system work, we must question in good faith whether the future needs of society regarding medical manpower are presently being well served at the collegiate level. At one small liberal arts college noted for its premedical program, approximately seventy students identified themselves as premedical in the sophomore year and thirty-four entered medical school upon graduation. Are we screening out able candidates for medicine at the collegiate level?

There is general dissatisfaction among teachers, administrators, and students with existing premedical advisory systems. Faculty members are often too busy with teaching, research, and administrative duties. Non-teaching counselors seldom have the direct contact with students that is possible to faculty advisors and are only indirectly familiar with course structure and educational problems. Students themselves are at fault for their disinterest in developing a satisfactory association with a particular member of the faculty, or they may be too busy or timid to do so. Administrative policies undermine efforts to provide satisfactory advising since promotions and salary increases reward research and teaching, not time spent advising students. Medical schools are at fault with their rigid curricula in basic sciences and for failing to advise premedical advisors as to changing patterns in medical education and practice.

Who is the best premedical advisor and what advisory system can be most helpful to students contemplating a medical career? The best advisors have traditionally been faculty members who have won the affection and respect of their students as teachers and researchers and who are able to find time for students. Because of increasing specialization of students and faculty, it appears inevitable that in both large and small universities more than one person will serve the premedical advisor function and that students will be guided and judged by committees.

I argue for the inclusion of physicians and medical educators on premedical advisory committees to give students an opportunity for early contact with physicians actively engaged in practice or medical education. I reject the argument that the physician as premedical advisor is special pleading in a liberal arts curriculum. One look about the campus indicates that specialization and professionalism have been with us for over two decades. During this time, there has been no shortage of graduate students in chemistry and physics. The changing nature of medical education, the increase in career opportunities, and the concept that medical education can begin in college must be communicated to the premedical advisors. The best way to do this is through physicians themselves. Doctors and medical educators need to be more visible on premedical advisory committees.

One pressing duty of the premedical advisory system is to advertise the career opportunities for women in medicine. In the 1960s less than 1 percent of each year's women college graduates applied to medical school. One reason women fail to show much interest in a career in medicine is that they are frequently counseled away from it (16). Also, collegiate women all too often receive a negative image of biomedical education from their campus environment. Admission committees need not feel, as some do, that women occupy the places that could be filled by men who are more likely to practice medicine. Studies show that the woman physician not only lives longer than her male counterpart, but may actually practice medicine longer. In fact, 95 percent of the female physicians in our two counties are still actively engaged in the delivery of medical care.[17]

The medical school needs a more clear-cut and direct line of communication to prospective premedical students. All too often, boys and girls are discouraged from seeking medical careers because they have less than an "A" in organic chemistry rather than because they lack the proper personal and humanitarian qualities. It would be helpful if the A.A.M.C. could take a more active role as premedical advisor in connection with its present function of providing college students with information about admission requirements. This could be done by establishing a regional representatives system to supplement the present advisory systems.

Multiple systems for medical school admission

Medical school faculties must begin to develop new criteria for selection of medical students. To induce such a change in faculty attitude, the number of first-year places will have to be increased and more financial support be made forthcoming for students. Rigid and inflexible basic science requirements at medical school and collegiate levels must also be relaxed to attract capable aspirants away from other careers. Present requirements in chemistry, physics, and mathematics need to be reviewed. Because of improved and diversified undergraduate curricula, students will continue to enter medical school with differing degrees of sophistication in their subjects. Decisions regarding a student's scientific credentials must be made in his best interests and with his career goal in mind. If we truly want to do what is best for each student, we will permit all incoming students to take examinations for advanced placement.

Advanced placement

Medical school admissions committees have paid little or no attention to the extensive experience of the colleges and universities that have been giving advanced placement to qualified secondary school graduates for more than ten years. At present, each medical school determines advanced placement independently and often on the basis of incomplete information. As a result, most medical students never receive advanced standing for material they have covered in college without being subjected to examinations reflecting strong departmental bias. A nationwide program of advanced placement would do much to eliminate the repetitiveness of course work between collegiate and medical curricula. An organization such as the Association of American Medical Colleges should strongly consider implementing a national advanced placement program.

The admissions committee is the most suitable body to determine advanced placement on the basis of achievement or examination, or both. Advanced placement should not be determined by an individual department. Under an enlightened system, those qualifying for advanced placement would have at least three options: (*a*) to advance in the continuum of medical education; (*b*) to pursue advanced science courses or research in their areas of qualifications and interests; or (*c*) take other courses such as computer analysis, economics or behavioral science.

If placement examination indicates that the student lacks the knowledge minimum to a basic science area, he may take a core course or intermediate course, depending on his ability and career goal. Disadvantaged students may find it necessary to take additional courses in the university before embarking on medical careers. Such programs should be carefully planned by the student, the medical school and the university. It is not unlikely that educationally handicapped students will require four to five years to negotiate the same medical curriculum that better prepared students complete in three to four years. In the ideal educational continuum, progress should be achievement-based, not time-based. What we are seeking is recognition by the admissions committee of variability in individual backgrounds and performance in certain aspects of the medical curriculum, especially the basic sciences. We also need gradations of basic science courses to fit the multiple career tracks in medicine.

A system of open admission

The proposition that medical schools adopt an open admissions policy for students with strong academic records is being put forth with increasing frequency. In the present context, open admission means no upper limit on numbers for qualified candidates. It is pointed out that such a procedure is more democratic and that it would bring to medicine a better representation of ethnic and racial groups than now exists in the medical profession. More particularly, the question is raised as to the ethics of restricting admission to medical schools when they have come to be more and more dependent upon federal and state support for their existence. Perhaps most important of all, open admissions would give each student who desired to study medicine the opportunity to, in Oliver Wendell Holmes's words, "show what he can do," and would avoid the tragic disappointment of the thousands of our young who are denied admission each year. Also important is the likelihood that open admissions would bring to medicine students with other than the predominantly middle-class backgrounds that now largely make up the medical school enrollment.

A change in admission policy of this magnitude would bring about tremendous changes in the medical schools. For example, instead of having a carefully selected student body attending small classes and a low attrition rate, medical schools would have to find ways to handle two to three times the present number of students. Undoubtedly, this would mean larger classes and the necessity for developing new ways of clinical teaching.

Obviously, such an undertaking could not be entered into lightly and without considerable study on its probable impact. Nevertheless, since the pressures for such a change in policy will undoubtedly grow, it would be well to study this matter in considerable depth. Therefore, it would be advisable to mount a major study under the aegis of a responsible body such as the Institute of Medicine of the National Academy of Sciences or the National Science Foundation, or both, to study this concept in depth and to weigh all the implications for both collegiate and medical education as well as for the practice of medicine.

The admissions committee

The admissions committee, a true reflector of faculty opinion and attitude, is rightly regarded as the most important and powerful committee in most medical schools. Most admission committees continue to be heavily weighted toward the basic sciences. Because of this and surely without intention, the criteria for admission to medical school have become unduly rigid. Similarly, because few basic scientists are either knowledgeable about or engaged in the practice of clinical medicine, attention has not been directed toward the advantages to medicine that could be derived from admission of students who have attained collegiate excellence in fields outside of bioscience. It would help to add the fresh viewpoints to our admission committees that could be contributed by community health scientists, biomedical engineers, women, practicing physicians, students themselves, minority groups, and health consumers. Basically, however, changes in the selection process can only come about as a result of revised attitudes of medical faculties. They need to learn more about the educational process and to pay more attention to health care needs and emerging delivery systems. If they will then accept more responsibility for broader selection and training of the marvelous student talent that we know exists, we will indeed be able to produce the many kinds of doctors that will be needed for health care twenty years from now.

Author's recommendations

1. Membership of admissions committees should be more broadly based. It should include women, racial and ethnic representatives, and consumers of medical care.

2. Advanced standing should be made available to all qualified first-year medical students and determined by the medical school through the use of national examinations or other appropriate mechanisms.

3. A national premedical advisory system should be developed to improve effectiveness of the present collegiate advisory system.

4. A national study should be considered to examine the principle of an "open admissions" policy for all qualified applicants to medical school.

Coauthors' comments

Dr. Medearis:

Women in medicine. Little has been said in the proceedings which have led to the writing of this book, and thus little is in its content, about the role of women in medicine. It is appropriate for us to consider the matter under "admissions" because as medical education and medicine respond to the great need and just demand for cessation of discrimination against women, a very large number of qualified women will apply to medical schools and be accepted. Infusion of this talent will have a significant impact on medical education and then on medical care. In order to anticipate and to plan effectively, it is necessary to include women in all those groups who are to make decisions about admissions, faculty matters and curriculum matters, as well as in those groups who are to decide about the delivery of medical and health care. The extent and nature of the impact of this change cannot be fully anticipated. We must now prepare for it by making medical education and medical care adaptable to this need. The possible effects of this change must be explicitly considered in every deliberation concerning medical education, medical care and medical research.

Dr. Van der Kloot:

Alternate plans for admission. The medical school admissions committees have become one of the most powerful instruments in our society. Those applicants who pass this hurdle are almost certain to graduate from medical school, and then it is almost impossible to fail to step into a secure and lucrative position. The rejected applicants are cast away without appeal. I hope that a few of the new medical schools at least will refuse to place so much reliance in the committees' judgments, based as they are on fragmentary and sometimes inconsistent evidence.

Some schools might choose to admit a larger, less carefully screened group of students into a one year graduate program in medical sciences. At the end of this year those students who have satisfied the requirements could enter the second year of an M.D. program. The other students could be offered chances for further training in other health related professions.

This approach is much fairer for the applicant who is willing to directly demonstrate his competence to the faculty of medicine and would eliminate that small fraction of the present medical school classes who—despite the efforts of the admissions committees—are unsuited by intellect or by character for the practice of medicine. Medicine may be losing some students with the greatest potential for creativity because they lack the solid and consistent records of academic achievement that assure the admissions committee that they are making a solid selection.

References

1. "A.A.M.C. Program for the Expansion of Medical Education." *J. Med. Educ.* 46 (Feb. 1971): 105–115.
2. *A Report on Physician Manpower and Medical Education.* Chicago: American Medical Association, June 1971.
3. Stritter, F. T., Hutton, J. G., Jr., and Dube, W. F., "Study of U.S. Medical School Applicants, 1969–70." *J. Med. Educ.* 46 (1971): 25–41.
4. Wallach, M. S., and Wing, C. W., Jr., *The Talented Student.* New York: Holt, Rinehart and Winston, Inc., 1969.
5. A.A.M.C. Division of Basic Research, "Undergraduate Origin of Medical Students." *J. Med. Educ.* 36 (1961): 1318–1319.
6. A.A.M.C. Division of Basic Research, "Undergraduate Origin of Medical Students." *J. Med. Educ.* 40 (1965): 223–224.

7. Caughey, J. L., Jr., "Admissions to Medical School—A Horror Story for the 1970's." *Case Western Reserve Alumni Bulletin* 34 (1970): 4–5.

8. West, M. D., and Altenderfer, M. A., *How Medical Students Finance Their Education*. Washington, D.C.: U.S. Department of Health, Education, and Welfare, Public Health Service Publication No. 1336–1, 1965.

9. Smith, L. C. R., and Crocker, A. R., "How Medical Students Finance Their Education." *J. Med. Educ.* 46 (1971): 567–574.

10. Association of American Medical Colleges, "Financial Information for Medical Students," *1971–1972 Medical School Admission Requirements*. Washington, D.C.: A.A.M.C., 1971, pp. 28–37.

11. Caughey, J. L., "More Medical Students: The Need And Available Supply." *J.A.M.A.* 198 (1966): 179–181.

12. Funkenstein, D. H., "Implications of Rapid Social Changes in Universities and Medical Schools for the Education of Future Physicians." *J. Med. Educ.* 43 (1968): 433–454.

13. Page, R. G., "Impact of Changes in Premedical Education on Medical Education." *J. Med. Educ.* 43 (1968): 717–723.

14. *Survey of American Pathologists*. Thomas D. Kinney (Ed.). Baltimore: The Williams and Williams Co., 1966.

15. "The Advisory System," *Preparation for Medical Education in the Liberal Arts College*. Aura E. Severinghaus (Ed.). New York: McGraw-Hill, 1953, pp. 22–45.

16. Lopate, C., *Women in Medicine*. Baltimore: The Johns Hopkins Press, 1968, pp. 25–42.

17. Mathews, M. R., *Women Physicians in Training and Practice—A Study Based on Duke University and its Community*. Duke University Medical Center, Durham, N.C., Oct. 1968.

5. The content of undergraduate medical education

W. Gerald Austen, M.D., and
Thomas D. Kinney, M.D.

The traditional program in medical education gave the student two years of the basic sciences that underlie the practice of medicine and two years of experience with patients. The curriculum was built on the premise that it was essential for every student to acquire a certain definable body of knowledge in preparation for the practice of medicine. Theoretically, the medical school by offering such an all-purpose curriculum produced graduates familiar with every phase of medicine. It was the belief that this traditional body of knowledge served as an important unifying force in medicine, since it enabled all physicians, both general practitioners and clinical specialists, to understand disease processes in their patients and to discuss their patients' problems with other physicians. This curriculum was developed in response to suggestions made for educational reform by Abraham Flexner in 1910 (1). Until the end of World War II, this program worked fairly well. In the first two years, the subjects of anatomy, physiology, biochemistry, microbiology, pharmacology, and pathology were taught by a basic sciences faculty primarily interested in preparing the student for work in the hospital. In the last two years the clinical faculty prepared the student to begin the practice of medicine as soon as he graduated. He was usually not expected to take more than a year or two of graduate training.

Unfortunately, this curriculum tended over the years to become standardized and rigid. Very few medical faculties recognized a need to revise it even though the medical needs of society, the nature of medical practice, and the patterns of health care for which it had been developed had changed drastically. As early as 1925, Flexner warned against the danger of standardization of the curriculum: "The desire to stamp out unfit medical schools has also operated to strengthen regimentation. . . . Our present fetters were therefore forged in order to compel wretched medical schools to give unfit medical students a better training. Now that the end has been measurably accomplished, the means have become a fetish, blocking further improvement" (2).

During recent decades attempts to familiarize the student with the rapidly growing body of medical and scientific knowledge have had several unfortunate consequences. Prescribed courses have monopolized his time and deprived him of the opportunity to indulge his personal intellectual preferences and capabilities. His learning procedures have tended to become stereotyped, rigid, and alien to independent and creative thought.

Perhaps the most serious consequence of the rigid time scheduling and the attempt to teach too much about too many things was the student's failure to develop and mature in critical scientific attitudes. With little incentive to question the reliability of material he was expected to learn, he tended to memorize rather than to cultivate the inquiring mind essential to a productive life in the practice of medicine.

The traditional curriculum also was too inflexible to cope with the diversity of careers that were opening to graduates of medical schools. As our society changes, new kinds of doctors with different skills are needed. Our increasing awareness of man-made diseases from our polluted environment and from the use of new and powerful drugs are obvious examples of new fields needing well trained experts. Numerous others such as genetics and the behavioral sciences could be cited. Equally important is the need for all physicians to understand the structure, operation and goals of health care as it is and as it should be as well as the qualifications and functions of the specialized occupational groups needed to make it function. Future doctors must also develop an informed and sensitive appreciation of the patterns of culture in which they and their patients live.

In the last twenty-five years, striking changes have occurred in the faculties of most medical schools. The clinical faculty now consists in large part of full time scientist clinicians who, because of their scientific training, are competent to teach the basic science material immediately applicable to clinical practice. Usually done at the bedside, such teaching is eagerly accepted by the medical student because of its clear relevance to the patient and disease. The basic science faculty has greatly increased in number and is deeply involved in research. Its members are making discoveries that will be used by physicians of the future but may not yet be applicable to clinical practice. The subject matter they teach often reflects the research interests of basic science and their concern that students develop a scientific approach to the study of medicine. The result is that the basic sciences are taught better than ever before, but their subject matter is frequently far removed from clinical medicine.

The change from teaching applied basic science to teaching the operation of biological systems without regard to their application to medicine has created a problem for the student in the first two years of medical school. He does not understand how a doctor functions. He does not know what knowledge will be useful to him as a physician. He does not appreciate that the training of the doctor who is going to apply what he has learned to the care of patients must be different from the training of the doctor who will try to add to the store of knowledge through research. He frequently looks upon the basic sciences as stumbling blocks on his way to becoming a doctor and only studies them to qualify for work in the hospital, not to master the subjects for future use.

The teaching of basic science is further complicated by the problem of finding ways to deal effectively with the steady increase of scientific knowledge relating to medicine. A generation ago the student left medical school with a body of knowledge that was not technically obsolete for twenty years, but today much of the information he acquires is obsolete before he completes his residency. It is no longer valid to assume that it is either necessary or possible for medical students to become equally well informed in all branches of medicine. Much of what is learned during the preclinical years is usually forgotten during the clinical years unless the student has the unusual experience of returning to a subject, and this is virtually impossible under the stringent time schedules pervading the traditional medical school curriculum.

The only practical solution is to prepare each student so that he will be able to acquire new scientific information when he needs it. This means that he must learn to evaluate critically the worth of new information as well as its applicability to the problem at hand. In short, the basic science experience should be designed to help the student develop the ability to ask questions and to answer them, and to acquire something more than a collection of facts that are likely to be outmoded in a short time.

The clinical sciences also have their problems. In most schools, they are still taught in the traditional way as a separate entity following completion of the basic science requirements. Numerous attempts have been made to interdigitate them with the basic sciences, but this has rarely been accomplished to any degree. In addition, the clinical sciences have been slow to respond to the rapid advances that have occurred in medicine, not only as to content but also as to approach.

Perhaps the greatest deficiency in clinical science teaching is the failure to allow for the fact that almost all medical graduates nowadays proceed to at least three, and more often four to six, years of postgraduate training. Also, many students now decide on a specialty relatively early in their careers. The clinical curriculum should therefore be flexible enough for the student to include course content that is preliminary to rather than the same as that he will receive during residency training.

All of the factors mentioned point up the need for faculties of medical schools to develop and maintain a continuing concern for the content of the curriculum. With needs and concepts of health care changing so rapidly, it is unrealistic to insist that the medical curriculum remain static. Medical schools that do so will abrogate their responsibility to the society they should serve.

Curriculum planning

The faculty of a U.S. medical school that undertakes to revise a curriculum begins with certain advantages almost unique in our educational world. Its student body is exceptionally able. It usually has a very favorable student-faculty ratio, and in comparison with other parts of the university, relatively good resources. Furthermore, one of the most valuable assets of America's medical schools is their traditional freedom to experiment—to revise curricula, shift goals, or modify admission criteria with few restraints other than their own judgment. This freedom is either nonexistent or severely restricted in other parts of the world. In an era when government is taking increasing responsibility for health education and care, this freedom is to be cherished and exercised wisely.

American medical schools are in a position to devise well controlled educational experiments that will not only improve medical education but serve as models for the whole university system. Because schools vary as to faculty and students, physical plant, areas of special concern, traditions, aspirations, sources of support and relative strengths of different disciplines, it can be expected that each school will revise its curriculum to suit its own particular needs. Such diversity is to be prized. If each school does develop a curriculum with its own stamp of originality, there will be less tendency for American medical education to fall again into rigid, standardized patterns as it did in response to the Flexner report of 1910. It would be naive to assume, however, that medical school curricular reform is an easy matter. Almost every school that has tried such reform has found great difficulty in devising a satisfactory method of approach. Although the faculty and student body may readily agree to the need for revision, for more coordination between courses, more electives and greater flexibility, their consensus and camaraderie may begin to disintegrate at the first consideration of which courses will give way to free time for electives, what body of information is essential and who is to determine its specific content. The viewpoints presented are difficult to resolve. The department chairmen understandably defend the boundaries of their disciplines and lay claim to what they consider reasonable hours of teaching time. The questions of who should be on the curriculum committee—professors or instructors—and in what proportion are quickly raised. The extent of student involvement is always difficult to determine. The politics of curriculum revision are real and directly influence the nature of the final product.

Nevertheless, to be successful, a new curriculum must have the support and understanding of the faculty. This can best be achieved by involving the entire faculty in the process. This responsibility should not be the prerogative of separate departments, but should be assigned to a series of subject or program committees representing the faculty as a whole. The concept that the curriculum belongs to the entire faculty and not to individual departments has had wide acceptance in the schools that have been most successful in devising new educational programs. When planning is left to departments, there is the very real danger that the curriculum will be fragmented and poorly coordinated. When planning is done by groups of faculty members with varying experiences and disciplines the result is usually a much broader and better coordinated curriculum with less overlap and duplication of teaching effort.

The criteria for membership on curriculum committees should be demonstrated interest in teaching, imagination, reasonableness, and high standards of scholarship. Most important of all perhaps, the committee member should have the ability to maintain detachment, to base his judgment on what is best for the student and for the school not on what is best for his department or discipline. Of special importance is his willingness to make a commitment of time, both for regular attendance at curriculum committee meetings and for studying in depth the problems under consideration.

Perhaps the most important members of the curriculum committee are the students. Not only do the students have the greatest stake in the development of a satisfactory curriculum but they are in a unique position to contribute to its development because they have had recent exposure to the premedical component and are apt to be more responsive than faculty to the changing societal expectations of their generation and to the needs of the consumers of medical care. Even though students often do not have the perspective regarding the total content of the curriculum that a thoughtful faculty member should have, their opinions should be carefully considered and whenever possible, their suggestions should be incorporated into the curriculum.

The faculty should be aware of and make use of modern techniques for planning. It is desirable for the curriculum committee to have as a member or as an advisor an individual whose training has been in the field of education. To ignore the advances that have been made in pedagogy is to deprive the medical faculty of a highly applicable body of knowledge concerned with learning and teaching. To date, little use has been made of systems analysis and feedback, nor do many schools have any adequate inventory of faculty, physical and financial resources. More use should be made of the computer to plan effectively for new coursework and programs and for competent simulation of such programs to assess alternative plans.

It is surprising to note how slow most faculties are to take advantage of the advances that have been made in the field of audiovisual education. Techniques are now available to provide almost any kind of a learning experience for medical students. This is particularly true for presentation of fairly standardized material such as history taking, anatomical studies, laboratory tests, etc. Audiovisual teaching aids offer opportunities for independent study and are invaluable adjuncts to classroom and clinical teaching, yet very few faculties have insisted that the possibility of using them be at least considered for every course. Instead, the use of audiovisual material is being left to the option of each department. A more logical approach would be to appoint an expert in audiovisual techniques to the curriculum committee for consultation when courses are reviewed or initiated.

Any faculty group that concerns itself with developing a modern medical curriculum must be aware of and responsive to the tremendous improvements that have been made in the teaching of science in secondary schools and in college. That the scientific preparation of today's medical school applicant is much better than that of his predecessors is not generally recognized by medical educators, particularly basic science teachers. The quality of college education has also been altered by advanced placement and honors programs. Clearly, this upgrading of premedical education calls for a reconsideration of both admission requirements and of the entire medical curriculum. The challenge to the medical schools is to find ways to capitalize on the better preparation of their students. Serious consideration should be given to: (a) multiple entry points to the medical school, including advanced placement; (b) multiple pathways through medical school; (c) a reevaluation of the basic and clinical sciences to determine what is essential for the practice of medicine; and (d) development of programs adaptable to a variety of career goals.

Medical schools that have made radical changes in their curricula in recent years, have almost without exception given the student greater freedom and flexibility than is traditionally allowed. This freedom has enabled the student to utilize more fully the resources of the entire university to make a career decision early and plan his medical school years around it. It is significant that these new curricula while differing greatly in arrangement and content of course material, have been in the opinion of the faculties successful in meeting their objectives. The relative value of course content in each subject and in each school is impossible to judge but the suspicion arises that the common responsible denominator in successful curricula is not the course content, but freedom and flexibility for the student. When stimulated to take the initiative in his own education, the student enthusiastically seeks to acquire knowledge that he perceives as relevant to his personal goals in medicine.

The basic sciences

Curriculum reform in the basic sciences revolves around these fundamental questions: What are the basic sciences germane to the practice of medicine and why are they supposed to be more basic than other medical sciences? Just what are the responsibilities of our basic scientists as teachers? What is the scientific relevance of usefulness of the subject material when taught in a world radically different from the placid academic world of the past where research was the password to academic advancement?

It has already been emphasized that the increasing disparity between the amount of information available and the amount that any single individual can master demands greater flexibility in basic science requirements for students of medicine. To make it possible for the developing physician to learn how to obtain the scientific information whenever he needs it, the basic science experience, whatever its content, should force the student to learn and understand the experimental method. The basic medical scientists should be able to do this effectively, for it is in their laboratories that the experimental method is practiced with the greatest precision. It should be their responsibility to provide the environment which will nurture the desire to learn and use the experimental method.

How and when this goal is achieved is not as important as that it be done well, for without an evaluative approach to new findings the physician will not be able to keep pace with the increasing complexities of scientific medicine. Some students will do well in independent study whether it be traditional laboratory or clinical research or some other project requiring original thought and critical evaluation. Others will find it more rewarding to make a significant commitment of time to a tutorial relationship with a basic scientist. Whatever the vehicle, experience in the practice of the experimental method will help the student learn to recognize sound criteria for reliability of information and to practice a healthy skepticism for dogma.

The basic science courses in most medical schools have already begun to overlap departmental lines as it has become evident that the principles of molecular, cellular, and systems biology are not unique to one discipline but together form a unifying bridge between all of the scientific disciplines and clinical specialities. What is needed for the future practice of medicine, therefore, is not so much detailed knowledge of the specific alterations of each disease process but an understanding of the fundamental biological concepts that are essential to an understanding of all disease processes.

If this concept is accepted, curricula should be designed to implement it to the fullest extent. Factual information and memory work should be kept to a minimum so that the student can spend his time learning to develop habits of independent thinking and scholarship to relate what he is learning to his future responsibilities. He should also be encouraged to maintain a high degree of motivation and to appreciate the importance of responsible professional attitudes.

If the curriculum can provide the student with an understanding of basic biological concepts as well as with habits of scientific thinking, there is no need to fear that specialization and its concomitant compartmentalization of medical knowledge will make communications difficult between physicians in the various specialities. Rather, the physicians who are the product of such medical curricula will communicate as scientists and scholars, secure in their understanding of the fundamental concepts of medical science.

In all probability, the future will see the elective courses become the keystone of the curriculum, and the success of a given curriculum will depend upon how well they are organized. The electives will provide the student with the opportunity to become acquainted with a variety of disciplines from which he can make a career choice. The elective system should then allow study in considerable depth in an area of particular appeal or survey study in several disciplines inherent to a chosen career.

Electives should be arranged so as to demand a rigorous scholarly effort. Their form should be determined by the technique of presentation which faculty experience has shown to be most effective, whether it be course work, laboratory experience, a research problem or a clerkship. Electives should offer a challenge to the faculty member who is interested in teaching, for they give him great freedom to present his ideas and to share his scientific and clinical experience with students.

Schools that offer a large number of elective courses have found that, given the opportunity, a student will almost always select a clinical elective over a basic science elective. This is disappointing to members of the basic science departments who hope that the students will return from their clinical experiences to study related basic material with a new perspective and with renewed interest. Even more disappointing has been the reluctance of students to avail themselves of science courses offered elsewhere in the university. The preference for clinical electives can be offset to some extent if clinical teachers strongly recommend basic science electives. In some institutions this is done by setting up special basic science programs or tracks based on the clinical departments' suggested lists of electives and programs best suited to different medical careers. For example, the department of obstetrics and gynecology might suggest that basic science electives for the prospective obstetrician could be the physiology of reproduction, endocrinology, cellular transport processes, ob-gyn pathology, abnormal growth and development, and exfoliate cytology.

In any event, the understandable lack of enthusiasm among medical students for basic science electives is likely to continue, and should be taken into account in the planning or revision of basic science curricula. The logical way to circumvent it is to make certain that the required courses include whatever basic science material is considered absolutely necessary to the practice of medicine.

Admittedly, this is difficult to determine. One effective gauge is to place students and faculty members into the setting of clinical clerkships and note what basic information the students find they must have to solve the patient problems they encounter. In effect, this constitutes a joint faculty-student research project, the clinical clerkship, to identify those areas of basic sciences without which it is impossible to obtain a thorough understanding of commonly encountered illness. Such an exercise quickly shows that the basic sciences needed for the practice of medicine include more than the traditional ones of anatomy, biochemistry, pathology, etc. It becomes clear that the student is dealing with problems of human behavior and aspects of the social sciences that relate to human health, and that for a conceptual understanding of certain phenomena, he needs to have an understanding of the physical sciences as well.

The clinical sciences

A more efficient and flexible approach to teaching the clinical sciences is needed to bring the new technology which is changing so rapidly into medical education. We must stimulate the student, excite him both by example and by our methods of teaching. We must adapt the many new and creative techniques involving the use of television, electronic simulation of clinical situations, computers, etc. The student must be allowed to be an active partner in the educational system. Didactic lectures have their value, but should be employed with considerable restraint. Pure memorization should be deemphasized and the student should be taught how to think. He should be placed in situations where he can set up a hypothesis and use basic knowledge and logical thought to arrive at an appropriate conclusion.

The clinical sciences have too frequently been taught in a rather haphazard fashion, with very little control from the medical school. Teachers are likely to be busy practitioners and/or researchers whose primary interest is not medical education but their own work. To be taught more effectively, the clinical sciences need a more rigorous definition of goals, constant reevaluation and change, and a clinical faculty with the time and interest to try individualized, flexible clinical education.

Some common experiences are undoubtedly necessary. All students must have the opportunity to understand and apply physiologic and bio-chemical principles to the patient, to examine the patient, take a history, make a diagnosis, and give appropriate treatment. They must understand the problems of growth and development. In addition, they must have experience with operative disease, the metabolic problems of the surgical patient, and the care of the critically ill postoperative patient. They must help to treat patients with psychiatric disease and develop some under-standing of psychology and psychiatry. They must have some under-standing of human reproduction. While there is no need for universally specific content in any of these areas, the experiences in common should include some exposure to actual patient problems and the introduction to one or more sub-areas of knowledge. Clerkships should probably be re-quired in medicine, pediatrics, surgery, psychiatry, and obstetrics, and all other clinical experiences should be elective.

It is essential that students be given experience with patients as early as possible. For the many to whom the basic sciences have been a hurdle to be surmounted en route to the clinical sciences that attracted them to medical school in the first place, early exposure to clinical problems is enormously exciting and a stimulus to improved interest and learning capacity. The exact timing of clinical exposure should be flexible and de-termined by the needs of specific schools and individual students.

As much as possible, additional disciplines should be included in all clinical courses. To teach cardiology, for example, without including cardiac surgery seems inefficient. Pertinent elements of the basic sciences should also be interjected wherever possible. Lectures and clinics should be combined efforts between the appropriate disciplines.

Each student should, with faculty advice, plan his career in a logical fashion with a strong emphasis on electives. Students heading for psychiatry may choose to take all their electives in psychiatry and the neurosciences. Those looking toward internal medicine may choose electives primarily in medicine and its subspecialities. Prospective surgeons may concentrate elective time in surgery and the surgical specialities including anesthesi-ology. Still other students may wish to be exposed to areas important to but not directly related to their field of interest. Obviously, there will be many possibilities for overlapping experiences consciously directed toward dif-ferent career goals.

Certain aspects of undergraduate and graduate medical education will have to be carried out in a setting other than the inpatient services of major teaching hospitals. This is particularly true for primary comprehensive care but also applies to the specialty fields. Outpatient facilities must be modernized and made more attractive and convenient for the patients. At the same time, cooperative efforts combining staff physician-teacher, undergraduate students and graduate students can be used to provide an ideal educational opportunity. The number of students per ambulatory care unit and per teacher will have to be kept small enough to insure effective health delivery. Care must be taken to find faculty particularly interested in this type of health care and in developing innovative educational opportunities directed toward improvement of the delivery system. Appropriate rewards for such faculty members must be created.

The teaching of the clinical sciences in medical school must, of course, interdigitate effectively with postgraduate clinical education, in which the medical school should take increasing interest. A properly programmed undergraduate clinical experience will make the traditional internship unnecessary. With early career planning and flexible programs in the clinical sciences, the student will be better prepared to handle postgraduate clinical and educational responsibilities.

The new medical school curricula are just beginning to have an impact on graduate medical education. Already, some medical schools are producing new physicians too advanced for the graduate programs currently being offered in our hospitals. These recent graduates would have no trouble bypassing the internship and entering directly into residency training in a specialty. They should not have to spend as much time in postgraduate training as is presently required and it is no longer tenable to require that residency programs extend for a fixed period of time. New kinds of residency programs are needed to allow for variations in course work of individual medical schools and in levels of competence among new M.D.'s.

When the last two years or less of medical school are largely elective, it is conceivable that they could be merged with individual postgraduate educational programs, making them part of the continuum of residency training. As suggested by the Millis Commission report (3), the internship would then lose its identity and be a part of the residency training program or of the third and fourth years of medical school amalgamated with the residency program. This would appreciably shorten the time required for graduate education in the traditional rigidly compartmentalized system.

The faculty at Duke University School of Medicine has recently devised experimental programs in the clinical departments to coordinate more closely the planning of undergraduate and graduate years. At present, these programs are limited to exceptional students. They vary in detail among the departments, but are alike in that each student is encouraged to think of the last two years in medical school and the first two postgraduate years as a continuum in which he has wide latitude in the arrangement of his work. These programs allow the student to construct a program that meets his special interests and needs, and permit him to progress at his own pace. Eligibility for advancement is determined by faculty evaluation, employing both subjective and objective criteria. The M.D. degree is awarded as soon as the third and fourth year requirements of the medical school curriculum have been met.

The goal of these programs is not primarily to shorten the medical educational process nor under any circumstances to reduce its quality. It is rather to modify present requirements for course sequence in the interest of overall career planning that is truly adaptable to individual talents and motivations, perhaps even to permit transfer of the advanced basic science requirements to the post internship or residency years if this is to the benefit of the individual student. For many students, these programs will cut six months to a year from the total time spent in medical school and residency training. It is too early to judge these programs fairly, but indications are that they will be widely accepted by the students and that in present or modified form they will fulfill their stated objectives.

Conclusion

It is important for medical education to establish evaluation procedures to determine whether or not the educational objectives of the curriculum are being met. This evaluation must include long term follow-up with appropriate feedback so that the school can analyze the careers of its graduates and their effectiveness in meeting the medical needs of society. Similarly, the performance of students in each step of the educational program must be evaluated in order to appropriately feed back and alter the preceding step. This is a process which we carry out to an extent subconsciously. We now need to do it in a more conscious, deliberate and thoughtful way.

The goal of the modern medical school should be to develop a curriculum that provides freedom for the student to find and pursue the type of career within medicine for which he has the greatest aptitude and interest. At the same time, the curriculum should be so designed that every graduate is able to fulfill the basic obligation of a physician—to assume the responsibility for the care of illness in a responsible manner. This is difficult to define in detail, but certainly should include: (*a*) the ability to take a medical history, conduct a complete physical examination and to recognize abnormal findings in both; (b) the ability to recognize and treat life threatening emergencies within the limits of the circumstances and equipment at hand; (c) the ability to diagnose and treat the most common illnesses affecting the population as a whole; (d) the ability to recognize his limitations and to recommend alternate sources of medical care; and (e) the ability to recognize and deal with social, environmental and economic constraints to obtaining appropriate medical service. Finally, the student should acquire enough familiarity with basic science to permit his continued scientific and intellectual growth.

The range of opportunities within medicine is already large and requires individuals with many different kinds of abilities, attitudes and sources of personal and professional satisfaction. Therefore, it can be expected that the graduates of most medical schools will proceed to careers that will differ widely, that an increasingly small number will be general practitioners and that a majority will specialize almost immediately in one of the medical or surgical specialities, in medical research or in medical administration. Because of this variation in career goals, the medical curriculum must be flexible enough to meet the needs of students with different social and educational backgrounds, interests and abilities, not just those who have excelled in basic sciences.

Conducting educational programs for the training of many varieties of physicians will undoubtedly be beyond the capability of all but the largest of our medical schools. Only a few can offer high quality clinical and basic science experiences in almost all disciplines. Because it will not be economical for each institution to develop broad teaching strengths in every area, reciprocal arrangements should be achieved to permit students to take electives in another school or even to transfer to obtain programs appropriate to their career goals.

Summary

Traditional curricula are not flexible enough to cope with the exponential explosion in biomedical knowledge, the changing pattern of higher education and the multiple career options now available in the biomedical field. New curricula are needed and American medical schools have the capability and the freedom to devise them. Because the complex politics of curriculum revision directly influence the nature of the final product, the process must have the support and understanding of the entire faculty. The aim of a modern medical curriculum should be to provide students with an understanding of scholarship and the application of scientific thinking to the solution of medical problems. In the basic sciences, it should teach the fundamental biological concepts that are essential to an understanding of all disease processes. In the clinical sciences, it should enable the student to study patients, to establish hypotheses and arrive at appropriate conclusions. A general familiarity with important clinical fields should be required rather than specific information. Elective courses will become the keystone of future medical curricula and the success of a given curriculum will depend largely upon how well the electives are organized. Essential to the educational process is the establishment of evaluation procedures to determine whether or not the educational objectives of the curriculum are being met; long-term feedback mechanisms must be provided.

Author's recommendations

1. The medical curriculum needs to be made flexible enough to cope with the tremendous increase in biomedical knowledge, the changing patterns of secondary and collegiate education and the multiple career options now available in the biomedical field.

2. American medical schools should make the most of their assets of an exceptionally able student body, relatively good resources, a favorable student-faculty ratio and above all, of their traditional freedom to devise controlled educational experiments.

3. Curriculum reform must be based on the concept that the curriculum belongs to the entire faculty and student body of a medical school.

4. Planning should be carried out by groups of faculty and students who approach the problems with sufficient detachment from a variety of experiences and disciplines.

5. The curriculum should provide for multiple entry points to medical school and a variety of tracks through medical school that can lead to different goals.

6. The science curriculum should provide an understanding of fundamental biological, behavioral, and social concepts that are essential to an understanding of health and disease.

7. Basic science experiences should be structured so as to develop an inquiring mind with the capacity to seek out, evaluate, and apply medical information as needed.

8. Medical students' common clinical experiences should be in medicine, surgery, pediatrics, psychiatry, and obstetrics. Well organized and rigorous elective courses should constitute the rest of the curriculum.

9. Evaluation procedures should be established to determine whether the educational objectives of the curriculum are being met. Long-term feedback studies must be provided.

Coauthor's comments

Dr. Medearis:

Education in ambulatory care. Education in primary / comprehensive care probably will have to be different from the education / training traditionally carried out on the inpatient services of major teaching hospitals. The major difference will be in the percent of patients seen by students, the percent of time any one patient is seen by students, and the number of students who can be taught in any one ambulatory care unit. The reasons for this stem largely from the idea, need, and demand that in ambulatory care the convenience and comfort of the patient must have a higher priority than that of the patient who is bedridden. The ambulatory patient has other important activities, and his health care must fit into a system of priorities. The bedridden patient's condition unfortunately precludes consideration of the patient's other activities; getting him well transcends them.

If the foregoing obtains, the net effect of this difference would be that medical school educational programs in ambulatory care would have to be affiliated with a larger number of ambulatory care programs (centers or units) than would be the case when these medical schools were providing educational and training opportunities concerned only, or in the main, with the bedridden patients. This will mean, in turn, meaningful, cooperative or integrated relationships between medical schools, regional hospitals, community hospitals, neighborhood health centers, and clinics.

If these differences are not worked out, it would seem to me that a high concentration of students occupying an undue proportion of time in individual visits or seeing a large percentage of all patients would so affect and alter health care delivery in an ambulatory care setting that the process would be less than ideal and thus make it less than ideal for education.

A special kind of faculty may have to be educated and trained. The physician delivering ambulatory care may need attributes and career patterns different from other faculty physicians. In concept, however, the task of providing a meaningful education for a student will continue to share the faculty member's time with significantly related activities in the laboratory or in the clinical research unit. For example, the one who is specially capable in teaching ambulatory care and providing an educational opportunity for students will also be spending a significant proportion of his time in actual delivery of ambulatory care and inquiring about it, activity not unlike the present occupation of faculty members.

Variation in the duration of educational tracks. A note is indicated on the length of education and training for physicians who choose different careers. It seems reasonable to presume that the educational program for some careers could be shorter than for others. Moreover, it is probable that as we develop better means for evaluating performance and consequently more capable in determining whether educational objectives have been achieved, we will find individuals who are able to complete their education sooner than others. It seems reasonable also that the education of the primary care physician might require less time than that of some other specialists, the academician, or the investigator. It would be so, however, only if the primary care physician could be provided with very much improved continuing education programs and an ongoing capacity to effectively relate to those disciplines (subspecialties) related to primary care.

References

1. Flexner, A., *Medical Education in the United States and Canada.* A Report to the Carnegie Foundation for the Advancement of Teaching. Bull. 4, Boston: Updyke, 1910.
2. Flexner, A., *Medical Education: A Comparative Study.* New York: The Macmillan Co., 1925.
3. *The Graduate Education of Physicians.* Report of the Citizens Commission on Graduate Medical Education, John S. Millis, Chairman, commissioned by the American Medical Association, Chicago: American Medical Association, 1966.

6. The education of biomedical scientists

William G. Van der Kloot, Ph.D.*

When this study was initiated, the preparation of a chapter on the training of investigators for the medical sciences and the promotion of a spirit of research and discovery in the medical schools seemed like the easiest of assignments. While there were gaps in opportunities and in coverage and openings for innovation and reform, the core of the enterprise was highly satisfactory. This success depended on the federal government, which had established programs to expand and fund the best of the programs in research training while also fostering innovation and experimentation.

In the last years, however, we have been taught a bitter lesson. Programs that took years to build can be undercut almost overnight. The resulting loss is more than a single project; the decline of confidence spreads like ripples in a pool. Today we are abruptly confronted with a generation of students who for a variety of psychological and sociological reasons, none really understood, tend to turn away from science as a satisfying and creative life work. The relative handful who retain interest can only view the future support of science as bleak and uncertain. Many students now in training programs supported by the federal government are unsure from month to month how long they will be able to continue. If they complete their training, they may well lack the resources to follow their craft. We have yet to feel the full force of the combined effects of disinterest and distrust on the education of medical scientists, but the results threaten to be profound. Confidence in the stock market is regained following a few weeks of rising prices and good business news; it is unlikely that the aftereffects of a bear market in science will be erased so easily.

It is all too easy to understand why both political leaders and young students have become disillusioned with some of the uses to which science has been put and with the failure in the United States to bring the benefits

* Many of the subjects raised in this chapter were discussed with Kenneth Clark, University of Rochester; Clifford Grobstein, University of California at San Diego; John Kinney, College of Physicians and Surgeons, Columbia University; Elliot Stellar, University of Pennsylvania; and James Wyngaarden, Duke University. The opinions expressed are those of the author.

of medical science to substantial segments of our population. Application has lagged and has been misdirected. But this is a failure in leadership and in enunciation of national purpose. It does not reflect on the validity or potential of the core of the enterprise. None of us can appreciate how deeply our lives have been transformed by science, nor can we foretell a future based on science without appearing to lapse into fantasy, hyperbole, or both. Surely, if men exist fifty years from now they will marvel at our ignorance. They will shake their heads almost unbelievingly when recalling the superstitions and half-truths with which we approached problems involving life and death. Historians interested in our era will applaud the explosion of biological knowledge that marked the 1950s and 60s, but they will be surprised at the lag we tolerated between the acquisition of knowledge and technological skills and their application to the vital tasks of medicine.

How much medical research should be done?

The federal government must provide the major support for medical research; the amount of investigation to be undertaken, and the number of scientists to be trained require high level political decisions. There are some who argue that research is a luxury and that our society, with its pressing and immediate problems, should contract its research commitments. There is no denying that research is always a speculation, but past performance and future prospects alike argue that medical research offers possibilities we scarcely can afford to ignore.

In the first place, medical research pays concrete rewards. As an example, consider only two advances in medical science whose consequences are easy to document in economic terms: the development of drugs to treat mental illness and tuberculosis. The introduction of these agents has resulted in a demonstrable decrease in hospitalization. On any given day in 1967 there were almost 315,000 fewer hospital patients than would have been anticipated if these drugs had not been available. The loss in productivity per year when this number of people are in the hospital amounts to $990 million. In 1967 the direct savings in hospital costs amounted to $921 million and roughly 3,000 physicians were freed for other assignments.* The total savings therefore was about $1.9 billion, a sum greater

---

* The calculation is based on 1955 rates of hospitalization for mental illness and TB extrapolated to the United States population of 1967. The cost of $21.36 / day per TB patient and $6.92 / day per mental health patient is used. Productivity losses were calculated using the per capita personal income for 1967 of $3,146. Data was from the *Statistical Abstract of the United States,* 1970.

than the investment in medical research for that year. There is no economic measure for lives prolonged or for freedom from psychiatric imprisonment.

Research moves into the unknown, so predictions are chancey, but the minimal achievements of biomedical research in the next decades can be forecast with some confidence. Methods are already available to decipher the detailed structure of the giant macromolecules that make up living systems and to verify these structures by synthesizing the molecules from simpler components. The way is open to know the major constituents of cells in their entirety. Techniques are now being developed to learn how the molecules join together to form the structures that do the work of the cell. From this point it is a fairly direct step to determine the alterations

Table 1. Comparison of R & D expenditures in industry and medicine

Industry	Total R & D funds as % new sales *
All manufacturing	4.2
Chemicals and allied fields	4.3
Machinery	4.3
Electrical equipment and communications	8.5
Aircraft and missiles	21.5
Professional and scientific instruments	5.4
Federal support of medical research	2.7 (calculated as in text)

* Adapted from National Science Foundation, *Reviews of Data on Science Resources: #17*. Washington, D.C., U.S. Government Printing Office, 1969.

produced by diseases affecting cellular function. We have the key to unravel the fundamental workings of cells and tissues. The question is how rapidly the key should be turned in the lock. The choice is clear. We can move rapidly to gain understanding, to exploit this potential for increasing health and longevity, or we can be content with a slower pace, accepting our afflictions with the stoicism of the past, pretending that they are inevitable. Of course, this is setting up an oversimplified choice. Everyone is for progress. The real question is, how rapidly can we afford to move?

One potential yardstick is how the investment in medical research and development compares with the sums spent in other fields. The research and development figures for major industries are given in Table 1 as the percentage of the net sales. They range from 4.2 to 21.5 percent (1). In 1968–69, the cost of health care in the United States was $60.3 billion (2), while in 1969, federal expenditures for medical R & D were $1.656 billion. The investment for R & D for health is only 2.7 percent, a poor showing indeed. (This percentage can be enlarged only slightly by adding the private support for medical research which pays for only about 10 percent of that done at the medical schools.)

Considering the importance of health, the known effectiveness of medical research and the opportunities now awaiting medical science, a well designed research and development program that costs 5 or even 10 percent of the health budget would not seem out of line. The size of the program should not be set as a fixed percentage of the health care expense, it should be based on a rational evaluation of what can be accomplished with the personnel and ideas available. For example, if a 5 percent R & D budget had been arbitrarily adopted, this would have meant $3.1 billion for 1970, compared to the present $1.6 billion. In fact, we probably could not spend that much extra money productively because we do not have a sufficient cadre of trained investigators. If we are going to make a reasonable commitment to health research, a major priority must be the stabilization and expansion of programs for training investigators.

> If science and technology were to founder or stagnate, many of our hopes would collapse. To the extent that we neglect this source of our greatness, and to the extent that we fail to preserve the conditions of openness and order that made our progress possible, we are living off the land of civilization without refertilizing it. . . . [Richard M. Nixon, October 5, 1968] [3]

Much of the training of biomedical investigators should go on at the university medical centers. They have the facilities and expertise for the task, and the proximity of research training is a powerful influence on the education of physicians.

> The practitioners of modern medicine must be alert, systematic, thorough, critically open-minded; they will get no such training from perfunctory teachers. Educationally, then, research is required at the medical faculty because only research will keep the teachers in condition. A non-productive school, conceivably up-to-date today, would be out-of-date tomorrow; its dead atmosphere would soon breathe unenlightened dogmatism. [Abraham Flexner] [4]

Research training of physicians

In 1968–69 there were almost 16,000 full-time clinical faculty members at American medical schools (5). Many of them spent a part of their time at research devoted toward advancing medical science. There were also research physicians, not included in this total figure, who worked part-time at medical schools, who were engaged in investigation at hospitals and laboratories not directly affiliated with medical schools, or who taught and did research in basic science departments in the medical schools. Increasing numbers of faculty will be needed if the supply of medical school graduates is to be increased. Therefore it is surprising to see that in most medical schools, research training is largely a peripheral activity.

Many medical students spend at least some time in research while still in school. Often this is during the summer when they are free from formal classwork and can join a research team for several months of concentrated effort. This experience is rarely without value. At the least, the student may discover that he has little aptitude for or enjoyment of investigation. At the best, a substantial piece of work can be accomplished by a student who is rapidly advancing in his ability to cope with new problems and to think like a scientist.

Although they often have definite long-term value, these summers usually involve real sacrifice by the student. He loses the opportunity to build up a nest egg towards the cost of the next school year. Great encouragement toward undertaking this particular educational commitment has been provided by the extremely modest ($600–$800) fellowships to medical students for summer research.

The medical schools that have succeeded in mounting substantial programs for summer investigation by their students have also been those that have turned out the largest number of graduates who later become members of medical school faculties. Unfortunately, there has been a drastic cutback in all funds for these summer fellowships. It is bound to have a serious effect on the supply of future investigators in medical science, and will also decrease the number of young physicians headed for careers in academic medicine. This will ultimately impair attempts to increase the number of students graduating from medical schools. There is a great need to revive support for summer research fellowships.

In many cases, a summer spent in a research laboratory is sufficient to get the student firmly interested in medical research. After that he needs the opportunity to learn more and to obtain further experience. This usually can be arranged, so long as his interests follow biological lines. Most medical schools now include elective periods at one or another step in their curricula, and the amount of time assigned to electives has been increasing. These periods give students an excellent opportunity for investigation. By using both summers and elective periods, some students are able to spend the better part of a year doing research as a part of the medical school curriculum. Their accomplishments during this time can be significant. Many of them produce one or more scientific papers.

A small percentage of these students become so enchanted with research during the first two years of medical school that they choose to spend an extra year in laboratory investigation, making the sacrifice of staying in medical school an extra year. Adding this year to summers and elective periods, these students may total two or more years of research experience while still enrolled as medical students. During their research year, students are usually supported by fellowships to help defray living expenses, and many schools waive tuition payments.

Undoubtedly, many students obtain excellent training and produce good science while doing research during medical school. Some are even able to produce work of the scope and quality usually required for a Ph.D. thesis. In my opinion, however, the usual haphazard and ad hoc arrangements often foster less than optimal training. Scientific investigation can be tremendously exciting, but the excitement is likely to be interspersed with long periods of failure and frustration. Successful scientists must have a compulsion to push on, to keep working until the problems and difficulties are overcome. Part of this drive must come from the investigator himself, but some is contributed by social pressures. Persistence and accomplishment are rewarded by the attainment of certain tangible goals. The setting up of a long-range goal is a central feature of Ph.D. training. Medical students who start research as a summer or part-time project are usually not offered a definite goal. Therefore, when the going gets rough they are apt to turn toward other interests. Some students spend each summer in a different branch of medical science, following the notion that progress will be smoother in each new area. Such a lack of long-term objectives can lead to a dilettante approach to medical science.

For this reason, medical schools should continue to experiment in the direction of formalizing research training opportunities and setting goals for their students. Several promising methods have already been tried. One is to offer the M.D. degree with honors to students who produce and write up a creditable piece of research. Another is to appoint a director at each school who can guide students interested in research, bringing them together so that they will acquire a group spirit and the sense of belonging to a program with definite aims. The director can also supervise the establishment of needed elective courses, seminars and lecture series. Ideally, the director of such a research training program should be a full-time and relatively senior member of the faculty with this as his major responsibility. It is the rare school at present that can afford this much investment in a sound program, even though it can develop one of the most important sources of new medical scientists and medical faculties of the future. This is the sort of activity that can profoundly influence the entire atmosphere in which medical students are educated. Funds to underwrite the decent training of medical students for careers in research are most urgently needed.

Proper training for research also requires time and facilities for advanced study in allied sciences. For example, many medical students interested in academic careers badly need further education in chemistry, physics, or mathematics. Under present arrangements, this is difficult to accomplish. Some ways to meet this need will be described later.

Postdoctoral training of physicians for research

In the academic year 1968–69 there were 4,966 postdoctoral trainees in clinical departments in medical schools (Table 2). The training was usually

Table 2. Numbers of trainees of different types at American * medical schools, 1968–69

Category	Number	Percent
Medical students	35,833	48.8
House officers	23,462	32.0
Basic science predoctorals	7,892	10.8
Basic science postdoctorals	1,200	1.6
Clinical science postdoctorals	4,966	6.8
	73,353	

* Adapted from American Medical Association, Council on Medical Education, "Medical Education in the United States 1968–1969." *JAMA* 210: 1455–1587, 1969.

based on a concentrated period of apprenticeship in a successful, ongoing research laboratory, sometimes interspersed with periods of further clinical training. The great majority of practicing medical researchers have been trained, in part at least, by this type of postdoctoral experience, so its value has been proven by long and extensive test.

Postdoctoral trainees with good previous experience are undoubtedly among the most productive segments of the scientific community. The combination of concentrated effort and youthful vigor with guidance from an established investigator makes for high productivity and accomplishment. An investment in postdoctoral training pays dividends in both scientific production and in education.

Nevertheless, there are some problems in the postdoctoral research training of physicians that are worth considering. First there is a tendency for isolation and over-specialization. A postdoctoral fellow usually belongs to a single laboratory, not to a school or a university. In fact, most universities scarcely acknowledge their existence, although even numerically, the post-doctoral fellows in the medical schools are noteworthy. For every 100 students in training at the medical schools, there are about seventeen postdoctoral fellows (Table 2). Perhaps schools should devise programs that will increase the chances for postdoctoral students in different labora-tories to get together in seminars and discussion groups, but so far as I know, no one has even talked to large numbers of postdoctoral fellows to discover their needs.

There may be a need for special, abbreviated courses for postdoctoral students. For example, many postdoctorals in biological sciences badly need the opportunity to learn more about mathematics and the physical and engineering sciences. Possibly, courses designed especially for them could fulfill these needs without distracting them too much from the central activity in the research laboratory. Again, this sort of development and experimentation depends upon adequate financing. A significant advance in this direction was the development of training grants by the National Insti-tute of General Medical Sciences. As originally conceived, the training grants would underwrite the creation of the entire environment needed for adequate research training as well as stipends for the trainees, but in recent years many of the grants have been stripped of all funds except those needed for direct fellowship support. This has prevented the innovation and experimentation that is so obviously needed.

Another serious problem in the training of research physicians is the continuity of their research involvement. Upon graduation from medical school, the young investigator may already have substantial scientific experience. He then undertakes several years of training as a house officer in the hospital. During this phase, all days and many nights are devoted to patient care and to the practice of clinical medicine. Meanwhile, science continues its headlong advance. When the young physician has completed his clinical training and returns to investigation he may be hopelessly out-of-date. Undoubtedly, there is a stage in training that must be mainly de-voted to the care of patients, and attempts to combine clinical training with extensive laboratory investigation are unlikely to be satisfactory. Some way should be arranged for future investigators to become house officers with adequate, vigilantly protected time to use the library and attend seminars so they can keep up with their fields. One day a week should be reserved for reading, discussion, and thought. Opportunities of this sort will become especially important now that numbers of M.D.–Ph.D. graduates are entering clinical training.

A final major concern is the role of the basic sciences in the postdoctoral training of the research physician. Before World War II it was common for young medical graduates who planned careers in clinical research to spend a year or two in a basic science department before returning to clinical investigation. The growth of large research groups in clinical departments has tended to attract young M.D.'s there for their postdoctoral training. Now, it is rare to find a young M.D. aspirant for clinical investigation who is working as a postdoctoral fellow in the basic science departments. Is this really a desirable situation? The movement of individuals from one discipline to another is a most effective way to transmit ideas and techniques. Irrespective of the nature of the problem, there is a different perspective to be found in basic science departments. Close acquaintance with this different approach may be valuable for the future clinical investigator. Both the education of clinical investigators and the flow of ideas within medical science could be greatly facilitated by a conscious resolution on the part of directors of clinical training programs to encourage their trainees to spend a year or two in a basic science department or in another department within the university.

The retraining of mature scientists is another aspect of postdoctoral training that needs intensive thought. Science is now moving so rapidly that some sort of intellectual retooling in mid-career may become a necessity; otherwise, too many investigators at relatively early stages fall behind and drift away from the bench. If suitable courses are developed for postdoctoral fellows, they might serve for the more senior members of the scientific community as well. In general, postdoctoral education has been too long the province of the individual laboratory. It must be recognized as a function of the university.

The training of Ph.D.'s

Perhaps the greatest single change in American medical schools over the past few decades has been the growth of Ph.D. training within their walls. These programs had to develop because the education of Ph.D. students is one of the requisites for a proper research environment in basic sciences. There is no substitute for the stimulus given a department by a group of questioning students with intense interest in science. The presence of a good Ph.D. program is a powerful—now almost indispensable—inducement to medical school teaching for outstanding basic scientists. The presence of graduate students also helps to establish the tone of scholarship and interest in basic mechanisms which distinguishes first-rate medical schools. At the present time, for every hundred M.D. candidates in medical schools, there are twenty-one graduate students in basic medical sciences (Table 2). Some idea of the range of interests of these trainees and the size of the faculty responsible for their education is given in Table 3.

The growth of Ph.D. programs in medical schools has been greatly stimulated by training grants provided by the Public Health Service (6). However, as was mentioned earlier, these funds have now been cut back;

Table 3. The number of doctorates awarded and the size of the medical school basic science faculties—1968 *

	Ph.D.'s awarded	Faculty size
Anatomy	118	1088
Biochemistry	246	1086
Microbiology	143	895
Pathology	29	1585
Pharmacology	131	827
Physiology	171	1023
Other	96	—
	934	6504

* Adapted from American Medical Association, Council on Medical Education, "Medical Education in the United States 1968–1969." *JAMA* 210: 1455–1587, 1969.

the future existence of training grants is in serious jeopardy. There is no way of telling how many programs will survive a drastic change in federal policies.

Programs for training Ph.D.'s

At this stage it is worth considering the nature of Ph.D. training, so that we can see more clearly how it can fit into the production of biomedical personnel. The Ph.D. has been widely and rightly criticized as an unsuitable prerequisite for a professor of creative writing, conversational French, or other fields in which alternate educational pathways to high levels of competence seem far more suitable. On the other hand, for advanced training in science the Ph.D. requirements set up a reasonable educational framework. After all, the major requirement for a Ph.D. is the writing and the defense of a thesis that demonstrates the candidate's ability to do significant scholarly work. The writing of the thesis constitutes the long-range goal that is needed to propel the developing scientist over the rough spots in his first major research effort.

There are other ancillary requirements for the Ph.D.: a certain minimum of coursework drawn from different fields, passing of a general examination in the field of major interest, and meeting other general requirements.

Nevertheless, the hallmark of Ph.D. programs is their flexibility compared to most educational pathways. They are flexible because it is assumed at the outset that the Ph.D. program for each individual student is unique. The degree represents a proved capacity for scholarship rather than the acquisition of a set body of knowledge, so requirements have changed fairly rapidly with changing circumstances. For example, most universities moved rather promptly to modify the Ph.D. foreign language requirements once it became clear that they were no longer relevant to the practice of modern science. At the same time, they have been quick to impose requirements in emerging areas like computer science.

A significant by-product of this flexibility is that new programs in new fields can be set up with a minimum time lag. To choose an example, a decade ago biomedical engineering really did not exist as a discipline. Thanks to the vision of a few individuals who sensed its potential, including some who could channel funds toward the development of training programs, biomedical engineering has developed into a substantial field that has already turned out some Ph.D.'s. Naturally enough there have been false steps and misguided ambitions along the way and many problems inherent to the education of such hybrids remain to be solved. My point is simply that the educational framework has been versatile enough to yield readily to new opportunities and challenges.

The medical school and Ph.D. training

The amount of Ph.D. training in medical schools. The Ph.D. training that goes on within the medical schools is a significant fraction, both in quantity and quality, of all Ph.D. training in the biological sciences. In 1968, there were 3,161 Ph.D.'s awarded in the biological sciences; 934 of these were trained in medical school graduate programs. In some fields like anatomy, pharmacology, and pathology, almost all of the graduate training is done within the medical school framework.

Does Ph.D. training belong in the medical schools? In spite of the importance of the Ph.D. training that has gone on at the medical schools, there has always been a certain uneasiness in the relationship. At many medical schools, Ph.D. students seem to be a distinctly secondary concern of the administration. Since Ph.D. training and good basic scientists seem almost inseparable, several newly established schools have decided to move both out of the medical school. One pattern is to transfer the basic sciences and their Ph.D. trainees to other divisions of the university and to have them come into the medical school for basic science teaching. This set-up appeals to many basic scientists, since it allows them to associate mainly with their fellow academic biologists and pay little attention to the problems of medicine. It also appeals to clinicians who are more or less disenchanted with science and feel that medical education has been distorted by a focus on irrelevant theory. Paradoxically, it also appeals to clinicians who enjoy and appreciate basic science so much that they are eager and willing to take responsibility for its teaching.

In sharp distinction to these views, I believe that the medical schools must retain both basic science faculty and Ph.D. training within their walls. Otherwise, they may dissipate the valuable atmosphere of adventurous inquiry and revert to schools for practitioners, rather than scholars, of medicine. There is also the danger that if the training of medical students becomes a secondary obligation to the basic science faculty, it will be treated as a stepchild and neglected as to standards and quality. Moreover, the movement of basic sciences away from the medical schools is sure to delay the clinical application of basic science discoveries. At a time when *relevance* is a popular slogan, it is worth reiterating that few occupations are more relevant to the solution of important human problems than the teaching of physicians.

If the basic science faculty and their graduate students are to be retained, many medical schools need to make major shifts in attitude and in administration. In most of the schools that I have visited, the facilities are controlled by the medical school administration which rarely has any idea of how many Ph.D. candidates are occupying their laboratories and classrooms, even though they may constitute more than a fifth of the student body. There seems to be no clearly assigned responsibility for providing the educational facilities for graduate students, and Ph.D. candidates are rarely provided with social amenities such as those arranged for medical students. Modern medical school administrations need to recognize the diversity and spread of their enterprise in order to provide a total education program including Ph.D. candidates, house officers, and postdoctoral fellows.

The existence of Ph.D. training in the medical school campus imposes difficulties as well as enrichment. Ph.D. training thrives at places where there is a critical mass of investigators with a common style for approaching problems, in other words, where there is a successful department. From the standpoint of the education of future physicians, the departmental organization of basic science seems undesirable; it tends to fragment rather than to unify, and to emphasize the foibles and enthusiasms of individual departments at the expense of the whole. On the other hand, Ph.D. training has thrived in strong departments and it is difficult to imagine any other setting as suitable for an appropriate research apprenticeship. To foster

Ph.D. training, therefore, some disciplinary framework or subdivision must be retained.

New training opportunities

Once the relations and the interdependence of M.D. and Ph.D. training in the medical center are recognized, possibilities for opening up new types of training become quite obvious. For example, many Ph.D.'s trained in basic science eventually settle in clinical departments, providing part of the manpower involved in clinical research projects. So far, no one has devised a way for these individuals to acquire a general background in medicine, although this would enable them to think more constructively about clinical problems. It might be useful, for example, for some schools to offer qualified Ph.D.'s a postdoctoral year with a series of clinical clerkships that would introduce fellows to the problems and approaches of medicine. Those successfully completing the program might be awarded an M.S. in Medical Science as certification. Such a background might produce far more creative members of clinical investigation teams than is possible with the present training.

Similarly, a few schools should try to develop two-year programs of medical training for highly qualified Ph.D.'s in biological science; licensure laws would have to be modified in order to make this possible. Some of these graduates would go on in medical research, but this need not be the sole aim of such programs. Many others would surely choose the full time practice of medicine, enriching the pool of physicians with their basic science experience and their maturity of purpose. The program recently begun at Miami can serve as a prototype to this approach.

M.D.-Ph.D. programs

One of the most interesting developments of the past few years has been the growth of programs leading to both the Ph.D. and the M.D. In 1968–69, there were 173 students in these M.D.-Ph.D. programs supported by the National Institutes of Health. So far, there are not enough graduates to be evaluated as to their effectiveness, so judgments must be personal. My feeling is that the programs will be highly successful because they are attracting extraordinarily talented candidates. Nevertheless, they are monuments to the wasteful rigidity of our academic structures, and should disappear as soon as we redesign our schools to meet the needs of today.

The programs were based on the confession that medical school curricula are too inflexible to allow interested students the chance to obtain additional courses and extensive research training without embarking on a second distinct program. They show us that the introductory doors to clinical medicine are closed to those who are not candidates for the M.D. degree. Neither proposition is defensible. In fact, I suggest that the decline of joint degree programs will be an index of success in establishing more effective programs for educating biomedical scientists.

Other sciences related to medicine

The incorporation of basic science departments as part of the structure has been one of the strengths of the medical schools, but there has been an unfortunate side effect that has actually limited the scientific basis of medicine. It has been difficult enough for the schools to support basic science departments in the traditional disciplines, and few have been able to incorporate more recently developed sciences no matter how obvious their relevance to medicine. It is the rare school that has a department of genetics; there are almost no departments of ecology, and only a few attempts have been made to build medical school departments of behavioral sciences or sociology. Nor has it been easy to pace development of good programs to the needs in biomedical engineering or in computer science. Basically, there is only one solution to this rapidly growing problem—to bring the medical schools into the universities. Traditionally, the medical school has been apart from the parent institution, often physically and almost always intellectually. Once this separation was tolerable, but it is now artifically limiting the dimensions of medicine. It is almost impossible for the isolated school to train students adequately for research careers in biomedical sciences, and the proper education of medical students requires more intellectual resources than any medical school by itself can provide. At this stage in history, the idea of establishing more hospital based or geographically isolated medical schools seems unreasonably short-sighted.

The reunification of the medical school with the university is especially pressing because the next revolution in medical practice may be more technological than scientific. New machinery may be more important than new insights, so it is important to bring new technology into contact with medical education. Let us consider some of the ways in which medical practice is likely to be influenced by technology over the next decade:

The range and reliability of chemical and physical measurements made on the patient will multiply. Methods are now being worked out to measure routinely and automatically concentrations of hormones and rate-limiting metabolites in the body. These measurements will largely replace reliance on second-order but analytically easy measurements such as blood-glucose, urea, and so forth. The automation of the analysis will also bring a new level of reliability to the data. This is critically important, because unreliable data simply generate more measurements and an explosive escalation in costs. At the same time, there will be a development of new biophysical measuring systems. Measurements of regional blood flows, responses to environmental changes, and the capacity to regulate and to preserve homeostasis will become standard tools, along with a battery of other new ways to estimate physiological function.

In a few years, the physician will be routinely confronted by a large body of reliable physical and chemical data about each patient. This information will have to be integrated with a detailed and readily-accessible history stored in central computer banks. The correlation and analysis of all of this data will be up to the physician. He will be aided in his diagnosis by suggestions from the computer system, but ultimately the judgment will be his. This means that physicians will need to have excellent training in the analysis of complicated systems involving a large number of variables. They must have an appreciation of quantitative interactions that is seldom called for in medical practice today. History has shown that it is wrong to think that advances in technology lead to a reduction in creative thought; almost invariably, they call for more. In my opinion, the most profound mistake the medical school faculties could make is to base educational plans on the idea that the practice of medicine in the future will be *less* scientific.

The impact of technology on therapy is also likely to be profound. The chronically ill will frequently be equipped with portable sensors and a computer that will constantly monitor threatened physiological function. The computer will be programmed to administer drugs as needed, or to promptly alert the patient and the hospital if there is a divergence from preestablished norms. Some patients will be trained to use their own nervous systems to alter function that strays away from normal limits, and the computer will serve to call these behavioral responses into play. Obviously, the brief samples that I have given here are only an indication of what is already possible and will shortly become routine practice. To achieve this transition and to take advantage of these opportunities as rapidly as possible, we must incorporate computer sciences and biomedical engineering into the medical schools.

Ph.D.'s and the delivery of medical service

There is at least one group of students who are studying for Ph.D. degrees but plan to use their skills for delivering clinical services. They are enrolled in the programs in clinical psychology. In 1967, there were 1,756 doctoral candidates supported by various federal agencies who were training for careers in clinical psychology (7). This compares with 1,415 residents in psychiatry and in child psychiatry. There are now seventy-four approved programs for training in clinical psychology. Almost all of these are based away from medical schools.

The usual training program has called for a somewhat modified Ph.D. program, with an emphasis on therapy, but a dissertation is also required. Recently, there has been an effort to move away from this formal allegiance to traditional criteria toward programs designed solely for the training of clinical personnel who will then be awarded the Doctor of Psychology degree (8). This seems a worthwhile development that might help to expand the number of trainees. With the tremendous national need for mental health personnel and the difficulty of increasing the supply of medical school graduates, this seems like a most reasonable way to help meet manpower requirements. Again this enterprise will prosper best when the medical school is brought into close cooperation with the rest of the university.

Clinical psychology is a model that should be pursued. There are also other areas in which programs might be set up, leading to the Ph.D. or to a new, roughly equivalent, degree that could provide well-trained, professional manpower for assisting in clinical care. For example, a few programs in clinical chemistry might be established to produce exceedingly well-trained chemists who could do an excellent job of directing hospital laboratories. Such a training program could also benefit from the abbreviated clinical exposure for Ph.D.'s that was mentioned before. Similarly, a few schools might set up programs in clinical physiology, to train individuals in specialties like respiratory physiology and electromyography.

In the next decades a whole new battery of specialists will be needed to policy our beleaguered environment and to use science to relieve us of the distasteful fruits of technology. Many of these environmental specialists will have to be trained in new Ph.D. programs in which certain medical schools are almost uniquely qualified to make a major contribution. Radiation and health physics is another area in which training is needed. The development of each of these fields could be mapped out by a high-level national committee responsible for establishing guide lines for education and for certification. Obviously, governmental or private funds would have to be provided to establish such programs.

With a severe limitation on the number of graduates coming from American medical schools, it would be interesting to see a serious study of whether a national program to produce Ph.D.'s in pathology, specifically trained for the professional pathological services needed by hospitals, could provide badly needed personnel and help to stabilize soaring costs.

Recommendations for funding

The overall question of the future growth and financing of graduate training has been studied in detail by the National Science Board (3). Their carefully documented recommendations on financing can be applied with only minor modifications to the training of biomedical scientists. They argue that federal support of education is especially important at the graduate level and that the federal government must gradually underwrite a significant, perhaps the major, share of the costs of graduate education. The training of future investigators and scholars cannot be left as a step-child to be supported indirectly by funds awarded for research or other purposes. In its own right, graduate education is vitally important for the nation's future. By 1980, it is anticipated that the cost of graduate education will be about 19.2 billion dollars, or 1.3 percent of the gross national product. To maintain a flexible approach, funding is recommended at six levels, ranging from the individual student to institutional grants to universities.

Summary

Our national effort in medical research and development is unrealistically low. Research is not a distraction nor a luxury. No other investment in medicine has yielded greater dividends in improved care. The expansion of medical research and development requires more investigators; their training is one of the prime obligations of the medical schools. This is a welcome responsibility, since the atmosphere of investigation is a vital quality in establishing the best environment for educating physicians. Therefore, the medical schools must remain deeply involved in Ph.D. training in science, and must take more seriously their role in postdoctoral training.

Present programs should be redesigned so there is a clearer focus in the training of research physicians and more flexibility at all levels between clinical training and investigation.

There is an urgent need to bring ecology, behavioral sciences, bioengineering, computation, and other areas of modern science to bear on the problems of medicine. The medical schools cannot build their own departments in each of these fields. Consequently the medical schools must be integrated into the universities to obtain the diversity needed for a flexible curriculum and innovative research.

The training of Ph.D.'s in clinical psychology might serve as a model for educating other doctoral students in areas where they can contribute to medical care. Such programs could be set up in clinical physiology, laboratory medicine, and cellular pathology.

Author's recommendations

1. Medical research has a proven ability to bring about vast improvements in health care and has more than paid for itself through savings in medical costs and in human productivity. It is wrong to think that research is supported at the expense of health care delivery; in fact, with our present knowledge we can never provide optimal care. Medical research is now seriously under-funded, not only in terms of its potential for improving the lot of mankind but even in comparison with the research and development expenditures in other far less critical parts of the economy. Funding for research and for the training of investigators in all of the sciences allied to medicine should be substantially expanded. The level should reflect high national aspirations and a reasoned evaluation of the sums that can be used effectively.

2. Medical schools must reintegrate with the universities to bring a wider range of sciences to bear on the problems of health.

3. The education of investigators is a major function of the health sciences school. Research training for M.D.'s should include a substantial research experience that emphasizes continuity of effort and the production of a significant piece of independent research. Ph.D. students in fields related to medicine should be given the opportunity to learn some clinical medicine, so they can contribute effectively to investigations of disease processes.

4. Efforts should be made to establish and to expand doctoral programs to train specialists in clinical physiology, laboratory medicine, cellular pathology and in other areas where Ph.D.'s could contribute directly to health care.

References

1. National Science Foundation, *Reviews of Data on Science Resources: #17.* Washington, D.C.: U.S. Government Printing Office, 1969.
2. *The New York Times.* Oct. 30, 1970, p. 16
3. National Science Board 1969, *Toward a Public Policy for Graduate Education in the Sciences.* Washingtton, D.C., U.S. Government Printing Office, 1969.
4. Flexner, A., *Medical Education in the United States and Canada.* A Report to the Carnegie Foundation for the Advancement of Teaching. Bull. 4. Boston: Updyke, 1910, 346 pp.

5. American Medical Association, Council on Medical Education, "Medical Education in the United States 1968–1969." *JAMA* 210 (1969): 1455–1587.

6. U.S. Department of Health, Education, and Welfare. *Effects of NIGMS Training Programs on Graduate Education in the Biomedical Sciences.* Washington, D.C.: U.S. Government Printing Office, 1969, 93 pp.

7. American Psychological Society, "APA Approved Doctoral Programs in Clinical and in Counseling Psychology." *Amer. Psych.* 24 (1969): 947–948.

8. Peterson, D. R., "The Doctor of Psychology Program at the University of Illinois." *Amer. Psych.* 23 (1968): 511–516.

7. The future of graduate medical education

William G. Anlyan, M.D.*

Before considering what the future objectives of graduate medical education should be, it is well to review the nature of graduate medical education in the past. In the late 1800s medical education in America was a conglomerate of British and German traditions imported by men like Welch, Osler and Halsted. It was centered in hospitals like The Johns Hopkins and Massachusetts General or conducted as a strictly proprietary enterprise. At that time, Lowell at Harvard and Welch at Hopkins were raising questions about medical education. They recognized its need for a firm and solid scientific footing. Osler was the leading proponent of patient-oriented teaching, and Halsted introduced the residency system, patterned after the German apprectice-professor relationship.

The impact of the Flexner Report in 1910 introduced basic sciences into the training of physicians and the practice of medicine. This marriage of science and medicine upgraded medical education at all levels and ultimately eliminated the weaker schools. By the 1930s, the undergraduate educational pattern was well established along the line of Osler's model at Hopkins. In contrast, the Halstedian residency system retained a loose apprenticeship character with requirements varying from discipline to

* Much of the thinking in this chapter was developed during a series of meetings with the distinguished scientists and medical educators named below. Its content and specific conclusions, however, are the sole responsibility of the author.

Dr. W. Gerald Austen, Professor and Chairman of Surgery at Massachusetts General Hospital; Dr. John C. Beck, Professor of Medicine and Director of Department of Experimental Medicine at McGill University; Dr. Howard H. Hiatt, Professor of Medicine and Physician-in-Chief, Beth-Israel Hospital; Dr. Thomas D. Kinney, Professor and Chairman of Pathology, Director of Medical and Allied Health Education, at Duke University Medical Center; Dr. Robert B. Livingston, Professor and Chairman of Neurosciences at the University of California, San Diego; Dr. Donald N. Medearis, Jr., Dean of the University of Pittsburgh School of Medicine; Dr. Kenneth J. Ryan, Professor and Chairman of Reproductive Biology at Case Western Reserve University; Dr. Leon Eisenberg, Professor of Psychiatry at the Massachusetts General Hospital; Dr. Colin M. McLeod, President, Oklahoma Medical Research Foundation; Dr. John H. Knowles, General Director of the Massachusetts General Hospital; and Dr. William D. Bradford, Associate Professor of Pathology at Duke.

discipline and institution to institution. No formal efforts to influence or assume responsibility for the graduate "training" period were made by the universities. Several reasons have been offered as to why institutional responsibility for graduate medical education did not develop. Among them are: (1) the fragmentary, proprietary nature of graduate medical education which required large numbers of professional and administrative personnel; (2) the expense; and (3) the location in hospitals which have been regarded as centers for the sick, not as parts of a university.

In this vacuum of responsibility for graduate medical education, there developed the present twenty-nine specialty examining boards at a national level. These boards, by and large, have performed an excellent service by setting minimum standards for residency programs and eliminating unqualified candidates for certification.

By the 1950s *medical education* could be depicted diagrammatically as a series of rigid educational and training compartments with one-way valves. Approximately fifteen or more years of professional life were consumed in getting through the system. The intelligent student completing high school did not have the option of advanced placement in college but was constrained by rigid admission criteria and graduation requirements for each compartment. College equivalent courses in high school were rare. The requirements for a B.S. or a B.A. degree were complicated by the requirements for admission to medical school. The student contemplating a career in medicine found very little leeway in the selection of college electives. There were rumors that liberal arts majors could get into medical school, but this seldom happened. It was apparent that those with the strongest bioscience background were the ones most likely to be admitted.

In medical school, the curriculum was equally rigid. There was very little free time, and the main aim was to give each medical student the basic information that would prepare him for a lifetime of practice. The information explosion and the rapid turnover of biomedical knowledge were not recognized, in part because the national expansion of our biomedical research effort under auspices of the National Institutes of Health had yet to be evolved. Except for minor trimmings, the product of the American medical school was stereotyped and was in large measure an undifferentiated "blast" form who would need a course of post-M.D. "training" before maturing into a real physician.

Following World War II, another compartment was added to the obstacle course of medical education. As part of our national and international obligations, two years of military service for all male M.D. graduates was decreed. In some instances, through special programs, such as the Berry Plan (1), an effort was made to specify the time in the student's training when the two years of military service would occur and to determine whether the work would or would not be related to his educational development.

Continuing education following residency training was not regarded as a must by any specialty group except the American Academy of General Practice (A.A.G.P.). A few specialty organizations, such as the American College of Surgeons, the American College of Physicians, and the American Society of Clinical Pathologists, should be credited with excellent programs in continuing education. The involvement of academic institutions in continuing education was sporadic; it varied tremendously from institution to institution and from department to department. The individual practitioner, except for members of the A.A.G.P., was under no obligation to refurbish his information base in any substantive manner. Unfortunately, far too many attempted to survive a lifetime of practice on what they had learned by the end of residency training.

It was in this setting that imaginative changes in undergraduate medical education were introduced at what was then Western Reserve University in 1952. The relative merits of repackaging information by organ system versus discipline are beyond the prerogatives of this report. The effect of the Western Reserve curriculum on the rigidity of the continuum of medical education was important for several reasons: (1) it demonstrated that schools could break away from the dogma that there is only one way of teaching or learning in medical school; (2) it illustrated the benefits of the Hawthorne effect—faculty enthusiasm for education climbed as a new and different educational program was mounted; and (3) it encouraged other medical faculties to think about innovation and change in undergraduate medical education.

So began the era of experiment and change in undergraduate medical education that reached its peak in the 1960s and has given rise to the present continuum of medical education with maximum freedom for innovation by all the institutions and compartments involved.

The objectives of graduate medical education

The ultimate objective of medical education in the United States must be the better health of society. In this context, graduate medical education should not be viewed as a separate compartment but as a part of the continuum of medical education. Graduate medical education must remain flexible enough to educate for leadership in the multiple careers essential to our present and future health care systems.

The immediate objectives of graduate medical education are: (1) Education of medical students for practice; (2) Education of medical scientists and academicians, including clinical investigators; and (3) Education of professionals to administer components of health care systems.

Can a major part of the educational continuum be changed without making sure that its end products will fit newly developing systems for the delivery of health care? It should be borne in mind that with an educational system of fifteen-plus years, changes initiated in 1972 will not affect the practice of medicine until 1987, at which time the educational continuum should be expected to dovetail smoothly with the health delivery system.

What this system will probably be in the 1980s has been ably described by Dr. Martin Cherkasky in the first chapter of this book. To summarize briefly, health care will be delivered in new sites, such as community centers. Doctors will practice more often in groups instead of alone and will be increasingly assisted by many varieties of auxiliary health personnel. There will be more ambulatory care and nursing home facilities. Medical schools will become more involved in the delivery of health care. More people will have prepayment and insurance coverage of medical costs, and some form of universal health insurance seems inevitable. Separate systems for private and nonprivate health care will no longer exist.

It seems certain that no one particular health delivery system will be suitable or even desirable for the entire country. A system fulfilling the needs of a large city population may not be appropriate for certain rural areas. Economically, the system should be one of universal, non-voluntary health insurance using a public-private approach.

Since it is our contention that every citizen should and must have access to the same quality of health care and because the economics involved are outside the scope of this discussion, the remainder of this chapter will be devoted to a description of health care delivery under a geographic time-availability system and the types of physicians needed to man it. Furthermore, the focus will be preponderantly on the physician and medical care.

A time-availability system for health delivery

A logical way to determine the most efficient manner in which to organize graduate training is to examine the kinds of medical care that will be required in each environment where it is most likely to be delivered. In this way, it should be possible to determine the setting in which a particular type of training can be most efficiently carried out. In the real world, the type of medical care obtainable is partly determined by the amount of time it takes to make contact with a physician after the onset of illness or trauma. Using this notion as a rough guide, a "time-availability" system could be worked out that would base the deployment and training of health manpower on the rapidity with which care could be provided for different categories of illness or accident.

Time availability rather than distance has been selected, since by the 1980s helicopter transportation of civilians could become a major form of transportation for those needing acute medical care. The time-availability system is applicable not only to rural areas but also to densely populated areas such as western midtown Manhattan.

Such a system would work in somewhat the following fashion:

Time available—3 to 5 minutes: For emergencies, such as drowning and other accidents requiring immediate resuscitation, the only care that could normally be expected would have to be given by someone in the immediate vicinity. Ideally, everyone should be acquainted with basic life-saving procedures as the result of universal "buddy-care" training in junior and senior high schools.

Time available—5 to 30 minutes: For trauma, accidents, and cardiopulmonary resuscitation, rescue squads with trained personnel and lifesaving equipment should be accessible within this period of time. Minor illnesses and accidents could be handled promptly by nursing and auxiliary health personnel in schools, industry, and neighborhood clinics.

Time available—1 hour maximum: With this much time to spare, patients should be able to reach the first level of physician care. Minimally, this should be available in a clinic with eight to ten assorted physicians in group practice. The clinic should share laboratory and emergency room facilities with a nearby 150-bed hospital, and the physician group should be directed by a primary care physician with a background in public health and the social sciences. Others in the group might be primary care physicians with a base in internal medicine or pediatrics and a part-time or full-time radiologist. Suggested educational programs for these physicians will be dealt with later in this chapter. Suffice it to say that each should be the product of an approved postdoctoral program, certified within his own discipline and with free access to the societies and colleges of his specialty.

Time available—1 to 2 hours: Here could begin the first level of specialty care, to be found in 250–500 bed hospitals. In addition to primary care physicians, the staff would include specialists in anesthesiology, cardiology, neurology, urology, orthopedics, ENT, etc. The physicians could be in multiple groups either by specialty or by inter-specialty groups.

Time available—2 to 5 hours: This should be the minimum time required to reach a major referral center such as a academic medical center or large urban hospital where subspecialists and the more recent types of complex care, such as cardiac surgery and kidney transplantation, would be available.

Ideally, the hospitals and physicians throughout the system would be part of an educational network. The system would function for patient care; it would also serve as the laboratory for the education of different types of physicians at various stages in the continuum as well as for training of nonphysician health personnel. The physicians themselves at all levels would have continuing education programs either at the academic medical center / large urban hospital or by visiting faculty. Another large modality will be modern communication technology through "hot lines," transmission of video X-ray images, EKG, EEG, and other physiologic parameters. Undoubtedly, transportation and communication will effect a major impact on the health care system of the future.

Education for new types of medical manpower for health care

The types of manpower needed to provided health care under the system just described would seem to be: (1) the primary care specialist; (2) the primary care subspecialist; (3) the specialist and subspecialist; and (4) the academician. Graduate education will be different for each.

The primary care specialist and subspecialist

Primary care specialists should function in minimum groups of eight to ten and would include physicians with graduate medical education in internal medicine, pediatrics, and obstetrics and office gynecology. Their educational programs should be tailored to individual needs and should entail about three years of postdoctoral work. No single individual can be a "pan-generalist" rendering competent medical care to all members of a family unit. Chapter 10 deals in greater detail with the future of "family practice."

Other new types of primary care specialists would include the emergency care subspecialist trained in acute and emergency room care, including acute cardiopulmonary resuscitation and minor surgery, and the medical director of the physican group with special education in public health, sociology, and economics.

The key to the optimal educational program for the primary care specialist is maximum flexibility for individual tailoring. The geographic needs of his area and the specific interests of the practitioner are two major variables that cannot be molded into a limited set of highly defined and rigidly controlled requirements. The latitude provided by individualized postdoctoral education would still be under scrutiny at certain checkpoints in the practice phase. For example, a program of continuing education would be essential; working in a group and not solo, the generalist and his performance in day-to-day patient care would be continually in the view of peers; the group practice and hospital would be a part of a service and educational network.

Primary care specialists would include the general internist and the general pediatrician as the matrix of group practice at the first level of care. The specialty boards in their respective disciplines should provide for such categories. Only part of the primary care specialist's graduate medical education would be obtained in a university hospital or its equivalent; a significant portion would be in affiliated community hospitals where common types of patient problems are the rule instead of the highly specialized situations seen in a university medical center. For the primary care internist or pediatrician, there might be a longer period of education in outpatient clinics, psychosomatic medicine, preventive care, and anticipatory guidance. The primary care physician in a specialty would not only be board-certified but would have equal opportunity for access to membership in the societies and colleges of his discipline. He would also be eligible for affiliated faculty appointments in an education network.

The specialist and subspecialist

The specialist and subspecialist will continue to be produced by present types of graduate educational programs. These programs embrace the latest developments and discoveries in bioscience and produce physicians highly motivated to seek a continuing relationship with an educational center and other continuing education opportunities through various modalities, including national organizations. However, the system does have some major faults, such as:

Uneven distribution among specialties. At present, there are not enough radiologists, pathologists, anesthesiologists, or otolaryngologists. Traditionally, the majority of our medical school graduates have been attracted to internal medicine, pediatrics, and surgery, leading to an over abundance of super-trained specialists in these fields. This distribution problem may gradually correct itself as medical school curricula provide more opportunities for electives in disciplines that were "frozen out" by the traditional curricula of the past as current trends of the economic market for these specialists attract more medical graduates; and as emerging leadership in these fields attains the degree of sophistication and specialization that has been characteristic of the departments of surgery, medicine, and pediatrics.

Uneven distribution of degree of specialization within a discipline. The point has already been made that one cannot man the health delivery system by having the entire graduate educational program geared for the super-specialist. It is equally hard to convince Department A in Institution X that it should stop producing cardiovascular surgeons and concentrate on the education of surgeons for primary care. The solution lies in persuading departments in the institution to recognize the need to use all of their affiliated hospitals and staffs to produce a spectrum of degrees of specialization.

Wasting time in teaching technical skills that can be carried out by allied health personnel. One example that has received a great deal of attention is that of the pediatrician who spends 71 percent of his time on functions that can be performed by a specially trained assistant (2). Whether the figure of 71 percent is correct or not will not be debated. Even if 30 percent were more appropriate, it would still be an utter waste of our scarce resources to incorporate such activities into the fifteen-plus year continuum of the medical education of a pediatrician.

The academician

The academician is, of course, essential to the continued production of physicians. With more than 1,000 faculty vacancies in the 102 existing medical schools in the nation, graduate education programs have a serious problem in trying to provide for expanding established schools and developing new schools. Medical academicians are not a homogeneous entity. In addition to the traditional disciplines, the faculty of the future may be classified as follows:

1. The *basic scientist* who has a major interface with the physical and engineering sciences in a university.

2. The *traditional basic scientist* whose major activities are within the department.

3. The *behavioral scientist* who has a major interface with the social sciences of a university.

4. The *clinical investigator* who has equal competence in a basic science discipline and in clinical science and whose educational and research activities are carried out in both areas.

5. The *traditional academic clinician* whose service, teaching and research activities are predominantly in one department.

6. The *clinician* concerned with improving the delivery of health care whose major interface is directed to hospitals and clinics outside the perimeter of the academic medical center. Health services research, computer applications, affiliations with schools of business management, joint appointments with departments of statistics, economics, and sociology are some of the features of this new breed.

Not all academic medical centers and their affiliated hospital programs can nurture all of these programs. It is more important for each institution to take stock of its resources and offer a selected number of educational programs of a high quality level than to espouse mediocrity across the board.

Changes in the present system of graduate medical education

What of the future of the continuum of medical education? What changes should be effected? First we need to recognize all of medical education as a continuum and then proceed to break down the existing barriers between the different educational compartments. The rigidity of the time sequence should be eliminated so that for particular careers in biomedicine, certain students can go through the continuum in less than fifteen-plus years after high school; others, particularly those who will spend their lifetimes in academic institutions, can mix the final phase of their formal education with the beginning of faculty responsibilities.

It is perfectly conceivable that in certain medical schools the traditional third and fourth years can and should be amalgamated with residency training. This would be possible in those schools where the last two years are on an elective or selective basis. At the same time, as suggested by the Millis Commission Report (3), the internship should be phased out and become part of the residency training program. Such an amalgamation of the third and fourth years with the residency program may afford the opportunity to shorten this span of the continuum more than has been possible in the past rigid, compartmentalized structure.

Continuing medical education should become a necessary part of the continuum. All graduates should be required to subscribe to an approved form of self-renewal. There is widespread recognition that continuing education can be effected in many different ways. To maintain certification, the individual would have to participate in such a continuing education program. The increasing use of the Weed (4) problem-oriented record in all hospitals and clinics will provide an important tool for self-assessment as well as peer review both internally and externally. Other important self-assessment programs on a voluntary basis have been developed by some of the specialty colleges, such as the American College of Physicians and the American College of Surgeons. The author favors a firm plan limiting licensure to a five-year period, renewable on evidence by peer review of continuing adequacy. The most important data base to examine may be the "track record" of the physician as retrieved from the computerized problem-oriented record of his patients.

Finally, the total continuum of medical education should come under the scrutiny of one coordinate body. The present proposal of the American Medical Association and the Association of American Medical Colleges for an expanded liaison committee on medical education to accredit graduate medical education programs has many highly desirable features. Such a committee should include adequate representation from the American Board of Medical Specialties, the American Hospital Association, and the appropriate specialty societies.

The university and its medical center must assume the collective responsibility for quality and quantity control of graduate medical education. A single clinical department should not alter its graduate programs autonomously but should be subject to review by the faculty as a whole. Implicitly, the likelihood for a coordinated institutional endeavor to meet health manpower needs would be greatly enhanced. Accreditation visits, previously limited to the content of undergraduate medical education, should be expanded to examine the institutional policies of graduate medical education. Specific specialty content would continue to remain the prerogative of current residency review committees which, in turn, would report to the expanded liaison committee on medical education. Under such an umbrella system of review, both within the institution and by national groups, the specialty boards should grant clinical departments a broader opportunity for innovation and experimentation in graduate medical education.

Author's recommendations

1. The post-M.D. phase of medical education must be a component of a flexible, noncompartmentalized continuum extending from college through a lifetime of continuing education. Where it is advantageous to the student, rearrangement should be permitted in sequencing of elective periods of medical school and initial post-M.D. training.

2. Graduate medical education should be predicated on the system of health care delivery within which physicians will operate. Suggested is a

time-availability system that would provide primary medical care within a maximum of one hour, secondary specialty care within two hours and tertiary subspecialty care within five hours. Emergency and health maintenance care would be provided in less than an hour by emergency squads, nurse practitioners, and other nonphysicians. National programs should be developed to train all citizens in self- and "buddy" care.

3. The training of primary care specialists should be carried out largely in community hospitals and clinics affiliated with a university.

4. Critical shortages in some disciplines in the medical school faculty call for special attention to education, development, and training programs for potential academicians in these areas.

5. Post-M.D. residency training programs should be developed in mind of the concept that periodic recertification will be mandatory. Mechanisms for recertification must be worked out.

6. Quality control and relative size of graduate programs should become part of the collective responsibility of the university and the faculty of the medical center, and not left solely to individual clinical departments.

7. The total continuum of medical education should come under the scrutiny of one coordinate body. The present proposal of the American Medical Association and the Association of American Medical Colleges for an expanded liaison committee on medical education to accredit graduate medical education programs has many highly desirable features.

Coauthors' comments

Dr. Austen:

The present policy related to the numbers of individuals accepted in postgraduate training programs is primarily related to the service needs of the individual programs. I feel that the number of trainees selected for each postgraduate program should be related to the educational opportunities available in that institution and also the national needs in that field. If additional service needs are required, these should be achieved with paramedical personnel. This is one mechanism, among many required, to begin to achieve national balance in the various medical disciplines.

Dr. Beck:

Patterns of graduate medical education in the 1980s may well be influenced by forces similar to those which have already changed patterns in Canada and continue to exert pressures on the traditional system. Over the past decade, the organizations exerting the greatest influence have been the Royal College of Physicians and Surgeons, the Association of Canadian Medical Colleges, the universities, and most recently the government. Since in Canada health is a provincial area of jurisdiction, the governmental forces have been exerted at the provincial level.

The group with the greatest early influence on graduate training was the Royal College. It took the initiative in establishing criteria for the graduate training of physicians, in accrediting hospitals, and in recommending that the universities be responsible for all medical education. It is interesting to note that the last mentioned received serious discussion as early as 1950 and that through the college's Committee on Psychiatry a request was actually made that all graduate training programs in this area be organized under university auspices. In addition, the college has served as the specialty certification body. Representing a host of specialties, it has, through the content and format of the examination procedures leading to certification, greatly affected the patterns of training of Canadian medical graduates.

In 1966, the college announced that by 1970 all nonaffiliated one-year programs (i.e. without fully approved residency training programs), would no longer be approved for training with the result that this undesirable type of training was rapidly eliminated. In 1969, a second step in a comparable direction was made when it was decided that only graduate training programs offering a full program of training would be approved, and that all those currently approved that offered just two or three years of training would be phased out by 1975 unless fully upgraded in the interim. Although it is frequently stated that the Royal College will only approve university-sponsored graduate training programs, this is not strictly correct. The net effect of all the requirements for approval, however, is that very few if any hospitals other than university teaching hospitals can fulfill all the requirements for approval. The Millis Report suggested that one of the reasons for recommending that non-university affiliated hospitals continue graduate training was because university programs did not have the space and facilities for all the residency programs necessary. Similar fears were expressed on the Canadian scene, but the 1965 *Census of Residents in Canadian Hospitals* * by Clarke, Fish, and Giles clearly indicated that university-sponsored programs in Canada could provide all of the residency slots necessary to train specialists needed in the nation.

The Association of Canadian Medical Colleges (A.C.M.C.), initially very reticent about becoming more involved in the graduate phase of medi-

* Clarke, G. G., Fish, D. G., and Giles, T. J. "A Census of Residents in Canadian Hospitals Approved for Training by the Royal College of Physicians and Surgeons of Canada, April 1965." *Canad. Med. Ass. J.* 94: 777–784, 1966.

cal education, now considers that these problems fall within its general terms of reference and that it should, therefore, become more concerned with residency training.

The universities in Canada were slow to recognize responsibilities in graduate medical education. This undoubtedly explains the reticence of the A.C.M.C., which is in essence a "deans' " club. The universities have been indirectly involved nevertheless through affiliated or university owned and operated hospitals. In most academic centers the members of clinical departments are responsible for extensive residency training programs, almost wholly conducted in hospital settings.

In Canada, the evolution of a comprehensive system of universally available medical care has advanced more rapidly than in the U.S.A. This development has been fostered and supported by cost-sharing arrangements between the federal (by providing enabling legislation) and the provincial governments, the latter being responsible for health services. Financing of this program has come about through insurance plans providing for the costs of hospital services, complemented initially by independent insurance plans providing payment for physicians' services. In this manner, universal coverage for hospital and physicians' services was established in all provinces of Canada by January 1, 1971. In the province of Quebec, the hospital insurance scheme began in 1961 and the salaries of all but the most senior trainees in the graduate medical education program were included in coverage for hospital services.

Quebec was the seventh of the ten provinces to adopt an insurance plan covering physicians' services. The plan was instituted on November 1, 1970, culminating a bitter dispute between the government and the medical specialists. The federal program supporting this phase dates from legislation passed in 1968. In this program, the federal government undertakes to contribute approximately half of the national average per capita cost to agencies of provincial governments through departments of health. In order to qualify for support, the provincial agency must provide comprehensive cover for all physicians' services. Benefits must be available to at least 90 percent of the population at the inception of the programs and must rise to include 95 percent of the population after five years. During temporary absences from Canada, citizens are entitled to benefits throughout the world. The plan must be administered on a nonprofit basis by a public authority accountable to government. Private insurance plans covering professional fees are prohibited. Provincial contributions to the cost of these plans are obtained through premiums according to schedules agreed upon between governments and professional organizations. Physicians may choose not to participate and their fees are not then restricted.

The number of doctors opting out of these plans, however, has been very small indeed. In some but not all provinces, participating physicians are permitted to charge fees exceeding insured benefits. Where adequate preparations had taken place in academic clinical departments, these schemes have only served to strengthen graduate training programs.

In the province of Quebec, more rapidly progressive changes have taken place in the graduate educational field. In the past, the Provincial College of Physicians and Surgeons was responsible for the registration of trainees in the health sciences. This college, equivalent to a state board, announced that commencing July 1, 1970 it would no longer recognize for graduate training any internship or residency position in Quebec hospitals unless the hospital was formally integrated into the residency training program of a university faculty of medicine. This decision gives the four medical school faculties the responsibility of inquiring into the residency training facilities of all specialties in university or university affiliated programs, as well as in any institution presently outside the university sphere seeking such affiliations. In one faculty of medicine (McGill), 120 senior faculty involved in thirty-one committees examined and prepared detailed training programs in fifteen major clinical disciplines. Since July of 1970, all house officers have been formally enrolled as postgraduate students of the universities (at McGill, Faculty of Graduate Studies and Research) and have followed a course of programmed study and professional activity designed to qualify them to become certified specialists at the end of four of the five mandatory years. For the faculties of medicine in Quebec, this was the first time in which each training program was examined in meticulous detail by a group of faculty peers. The plan has already proved a laudatory one. It is important to recognize that government, through its hospital insurance system, agrees to finance the number of trainees arrived at by the university, provincial college and governmental authorities, up to the time of completion of their training programs.

With increasing governmental support of graduate training as well as overall health care, there is a real danger that decisions influencing this training will be made by government or hospital administrators, neither of which is usually in a position to evaluate training opportunities or to decide on the number of trainees who may enter a given program. Both are influenced by the increasing demand for trained physicians and the counter-force of financial factors that may dictate reduction in the number of trainees in a given department or institution. Study of the level of financial support for trainees and recognizing their service function during their educational program is mandatory to a solution of one of the problems in graduate medical education.

Dr. Medearis:

The interface between the education of the pediatrician and that of the internist will vary, of course, depending upon whether that phase of their graduate education under consideration deals predominantly with specialization according to systems or diseases or with comprehensive and primary care of the infant or adult as a member of a family and the community. In the former, the interface will be at the consultation level and will depend upon the expertise the specialist is able to bring to the solution of a particular problem, one which is usually complicated and acute. Thus the internist and pediatrician and their students who are concerned with infectious disease or cardiology or endocrinology will focus on that subspecialty and relate to it within a context established by whether the patient is an infant or an adult. Such contacts between pediatricians and internists-to-be will be occasional and focused on the disease process. I do not see that our current educational programs have to be changed in regard to this matter. I do believe we must encourage directors of training grants and fellowship programs to include pediatrics and medicine, e.g., there should be a single infectious disease training grant encompassing all medical specialties, especially medicine and pediatrics.

In education relating to the delivery of primary comprehensive health care to infants and children or to adults, the interaction should be different. There are phases in the lifetime of a family when the services of one specialist are needed more often than those of another. The young family with infants and children will require medical expertise principally within the area of health care for their children. The pediatrician is the one most capable of caring for that family. In the history of man, infants and children have not been fortunate. There is not only a demand, there is an overwhelming need that society recognize that there must be amongst it persons whose overwhelming concern and capability is to insure the optimal development of the child. For these two reasons in the setting of the group practice or a neighborhood health center the family with young children should be cared for by a well-educated, well-trained pediatrician who has an internist, obstetrician, and psychiatrist within call when the need arises.

The medical and health care of families that requires the internist more frequently begins during the third and fourth decade where both internist and pediatrician are needed to give appropriate care to the adolescent. In order to provide adequately for the ambulatory health care of the family at this time, there must be a very close working relationship between the internist and pediatrician. Later in the life of the family the services of the internist will be most needed. Therefore, the internist is the appropriate and most highly qualified physician to care for the family when there are older children or none. If the health care of the family is provided by a family practitioner, he cannot adequately provide the advocacy role so necessary in psychosocial care problems, or in those instances especially relating to the medical care needs of the infant and child, nor can he provide the expertise of an internist or pediatrician.

Groups of families can probably be cared for best by groups of internists and pediatricians. In order to provide those educational opportunities that will enable students to learn how to operate within the interface between internist and pediatrician in the delivery of primary comprehensive care, it will be necessary to provide appropriate models. This can be done in neighborhood health centers, doctors' offices, and group practices where internists and pediatricians are working well together. In contrast, to learn the interaction of the two at the consultation level we need only to continue to provide the excellent specialty services now available in most university health centers. Again the idea is to provide excellence in health care delivery so as to provide an ideal model for the education of those professionals who will deliver health care.

In summary, the proposition is that an educational program in the delivery of primary / comprehensive care to families cannot be provided on the wards of university health centers; instead, pediatricians and internists will have to have their education in facilities and programs where they can deliver primary care together. The intent here is not to exclude the possibility that family practitioners could not be adequately educated and trained, nor that they could not provide excellent care; rather the intent is to establish which course seems to have greater promise and to pursue it.

Dr. Stead:

Medical schools and medical centers involved in education can be efficient units for producing a wide spectrum of medical manpower. Their primary output is people. They use research and patient service as tools to aid in the educational process. They are not, and cannot be, equally efficient producers of research or patient service. A patient involved in the teaching program may receive excellent medical care, but it is never given in the fastest manner for the lowest cost.

The necessary inefficiencies in terms of service of educational units must be appreciated when one is projecting extension of medical school services into units primarily designed for service. The cash flow through the health care unit is rarely great enough to finance both the faculty and the inefficiencies of the services when a large number of students and residents are present. To make the new unit an effective teaching unit, moneys must be found to pay for the educational costs. These moneys must approximate the sums paid for education in the university hospital or the education given in the peripheral unit will be of an inferior grade.

With the increase in the number of medical students, medical schools must decentralize, and the number of primary teaching units must expand. The keepers of the budget must be prepared for the new educational expenses which cannot be properly charged to the patient-care dollar.

The extrapolation of the teaching model and its necessary inefficiencies into all hospitals and clinics giving patient care would be prohibitively expensive and would mean that no sector of our society received efficient, low-cost health services. The Kaiser Permanente plan does not pay for the production of medical manpower. They are agreeable to their doctors spending a stipulated amount of time in the inefficient medical school shops, but they do not want to bring these inefficiencies into their own shop.

Medical educators attempting to relate to the community always try to export the student-intern-resident model. It is all they know. At Duke, Dr. E. Harvey Estes and his group have been developing clinical support systems—new mixes of men and machines—which can allow the doctor to function effectively in the community. We believe these new models can give better and cheaper health care than the student-intern-resident model. The educational units should not be expanded beyond the needs for trained medical manpower. The giving of health services is best separated from the educational units whenever possible. A system of rotation of personnel from the efficient service areas back through the inefficient educational units is desirable and practical. It is much cheaper than the conversion of every service unit into an educational unit. Every doctor in practice who interacts with the teaching hospital by working in it for a given period of time each year has separated his day into time spent in an inefficient educational unit and time spent in a more efficient service unit.

References

1. Department of Defense, *Berry Plan—Information Bulletin.* Washington, D.C.: U.S. Government Printing Office, 1970.
2. Silver, H. K., and Hecker, J. A., "The Pediatric Nurse Practitioner and the Child Health Associate: New Types of Health Professionals." *J. Med. Educ.* 45 (1970): 171–176.
3. *The Graduate Education of Physicians.* The report of the Citizens Commission on Graduate Medical Education, John S. Millis, Chairman, Chicago: American Medical Association, 1966.
4. Weed, L. L., *Medical Records, Medical Education, and Patient Care.* Cleveland: Case Western Reserve University Press, 1969, pp. 1–273.

8. Continuing medical education

John C. Beck, M.D.

The definition of continuing education requires a commitment to lifelong scholarship. This applies in clinical medicine, in particular, but also in other areas of the health professions; an obsolete physician-scientist is as great an economic and educational disaster as an obsolete practicing physician. For this commitment to be effective, the individual must be dedicated to continuous self-renewal, which requires the retention of curiosity, perseverance, initiative, and other qualities essential for learning. Efforts to project into the future are complicated by the realization that future programs of continuing education will inevitably be bound in with patterns of health care delivery yet to be evolved and defined. Several statements may be made which pinpoint the problem further.

The first is that a review of the methods currently used in continuing medical education clearly reveals a lack of consensus as to which methods are the best. Those in common use include personal contact between the practicing physician and the specialist consultant, attendance at scientific meetings, perusal of professional journals and other publications, seminars, audio and audiovisual tapes, postgraduate courses, visiting speakers at local medical society meetings, and TV broadcast conferences.

Second, the majority of these techniques are probably outmoded already, and through them we merely pay lip service to the necessity of continuing education for the practicing physician. This applies particularly to the postgraduate course, the visiting speaker at the local medical society meeting, audio and audiovisual tapes, the TV broadcast conference, and selected journal reading. They require no active participation and lack other ingredients essential to the pursuit of scholarship. Few of these models have been rigorously tested to see whether they alter the professional behavior of the physician.

Third, there are essentially three constituencies for continuing education in 1971. The first is the "distant" M.D. graduate; the second, the more recent M.D. who is five to ten years past the end of his graduate training; and the third group consists of the students now in training from collegiate through postgraduate levels. A solution to the problem of continuing education for each of these three constituencies is not easily arrived at. For the first group, the "distant" M.D. graduate, we will have to persist with the timeworn approach, hoping for further impact from modern educational technology now becoming available. An example that is meeting with increasing favor is the application of the computer to problem solving of a purely clinical type. New technology in the rapidly evolving audiovisual area will undoubtedly facilitate learning if it can be coupled with devices to evaluate the degree of actual reeducation. If rationally applied, the impact of newer patient data storage systems and their easy review by the so-called medical audit will substantially expand the self-educational potential of physicians in practice. The value of "self-assessment" programs, such as those sponsored by the American College of Physicians, remains unknown, but they may help these physicians to define their own particular areas of weakness. Practicing physicians, however, will be very difficult to retrieve for scholarly pursuit, and they will remain relatively uninfluenced by the increasingly favored concept of recertification.

A possible mechanism for influencing the second group of physicians, those five to ten years out of the educational system, is described as a "physician-in-residence" program. This has been attempted in a few narrow specialty areas, such as neurology, and is being tried at the moment in other specialty areas. This program, which is purely experimental, attempts to meet several objectives. The first would be to provide physicians primarily concerned with clinical care with recurrent time for thought and with constant intellectual challenge. A second objective would be for the development of models which would favor the reorganization of community medicine and which could eventually be transported from the university setting into the community.

As envisaged, the physician-in-residence would be a practicing physician who would relinquish his practice for one or several months per year and spend this time, initially, under the auspices of a university hospital. Participating physicians could combine in groups of twelve, for example, if a one-month stint were involved, so that the practice of the one who was away could be covered by his colleagues. At least two types of trial programs can be formulated. In fact, they are being seriously considered at the operational level. The first, in general internal medicine, would incorporate the physician-in-residence into the graduate training program of the department of medicine at the university hospital. There he would be given adequate time for reading and consultation and would actively participate in the organization of conferences. The second type would allow the physician to associate himself with a specialty group in a medical school or hospital.

In each of these systems the physician-in-residence, having selected a field of interest, could learn new concepts and new techniques, not passively but in active participation with the group for a significant period of time. He could then apply his new learning to practice. If general and specialty rotations were alternated, the physician could add diversity and fresh approaches to his improved competence for patient care, hopefully, and would be motivated to continuous scholarship.

If models such as these prove workable in the university hospital, it seems likely that they could be copied at the larger community hospitals with many benefits. Here the physician-in-residence could concern himself primarily with the patients hospitalized by his eleven other colleagues (using the one-month, twelve-physician model). He would see, evaluate, and discuss these patients with other members of the group. Two or three physicians-in-residence might work with physicians from the full-time staff; they might well have students and other health professionals as part of the total learning team. This physician-in-residence model in the community hospital would give participants an annual opportunity for refreshing the mind through reading and for the active pursuit of problems in general medicine in combination with teaching. It would also guarantee that the eleven other members of the group would have someone to debate with throughout the year and to depend upon to some extent when admitting patients to the hospital. Its weakness, of course, is that it is primarily hospital-based, but this particular disadvantage could be overcome by increasing the number of ambulatory care facilities. The financial implications of this program on an individual physician's earnings would have to be considered and budgeted for.

An alternative or complementary procedure, which theoretically might be equally effective, would be the planned rotation of university health center personnel to peripheral institutions for effective periods of time. Its disadvantage from the major hospitals' point of view would be the very real increase in faculty that would be required.

The final group, students in training, poses an entirely separate problem. Viewed as a whole, the output from our North American medical schools is good, so one of the major reasons for the rapid obsolescence of our graduates must be that we are not using them properly. At the end of training, they are being placed in an environment which is not intellectually satisfying to them. Clearly, some of the newer approaches, such as the physician's assistant program, might help to enrich that environment by giving to the physician another kind of role.

The importance of continuing education in the practice of medicine should first be stressed while future practitioners are still in medical school. It is here that professional habits of thought are initially acquired, and the majority of faculty members with whom the students come in contact are themselves aware of the importance of constantly updating their knowledge and skills. In this early phase of their careers, students are perhaps most receptive and sensitive to the views of their teachers. How can this fertile period be used to cultivate in students the habit of continuous renewal? How can they be helped to develop critical and durable qualities that will serve them in circumstances that cannot be anticipated? With the inculcation of these qualities as a major objective, educators must attempt to develop mechanisms for accomplishing it. It is crucial to emphasize constantly the dynamic nature of the practice of medicine, the delicate relationship between the relatively stable art and the rapidly changing science, the tentative nature of accepted tenets, and the fallacies of some beliefs that were widely accepted in the past.

With the realization that not all practitioners need or can profit by the same course or courses of study in a continuing education program, the program must be made as flexible as possible. The major concern of each, of course, is to expand his knowledge of the area in which he practices or performs services. Different programs will thus be required for different groups of practitioners within the same profession.

If time becomes available to physicians for renewal, how can we make sure that in the absence of a powerful stimulus it will be utilized for this purpose? Perhaps recertification or relicensure or limited licensure can serve as such a stimulus. The wisdom of ensuring continued competence of a practitioner after professional qualification is being increasingly recognized in other fields. In medicine, the real issue is what means can be employed to achieve this end. Existing mechanisms are quite inadequate for the task and have largely been centered about disciplinary action for professional misconduct, a control which operates only when advanced obsolescence has occurred. In our present system, the problem of maintaining competence is intensified by the isolation in which so many practitioners work. This makes it unlikely that any incompetence that exists will be discovered.

The technique most often considered for ensuring competence is periodic reexamination. One of the major defects of traditional examination systems, however, is their limited capacity for measuring many of the qualities which make for professional competence. Recently, the National Board of Medical Examiners and the American Board of Internal Medicine (A.B.I.M.) have collaborated in a program aimed at developing new evaluation instruments. These may have a major impact upon testing for factual knowledge and the components necessary for clinical competence. They involve the use of computer facilities for the storage of information concerning patients and the examinee's approach to the solution of the problems presented.

Increasing numbers of professional bodies concerned with the activities of health personnel are discussing recertification. Early in 1969, one of the most influential of these, A.B.I.M., formally adopted the principle of recertification and has notified all its subsequent certificants that in the future their certificate would be subject to renewal. Discussions were instituted between the A.B.I.M. and the American College of Physicians about the frequency of the recertification procedure, the mechanisms for recertification, and the organizations who should be responsible for this procedure. From these discussions it was decided that recertification in internal medicine is the responsibility of the A.B.I.M. since it is the original certifying body; also that recertification should take place no more frequently than every five years. The issue of whether recertification should be compulsory continues to be discussed. The *Report of the National Advisory Commission on Health Manpower* (U.S. Government Printing Office, 1967) advised against compulsory recertification and the present stance of the A.B.I.M. is that recertification should be regarded as an accolade and as such, an additional indication of competence.

Limited licensure, suggested as a mechanism for quality control, might also simplify the problem of guaranteeing continued competence. Such a procedure would limit the graduate of a medical school to practice in a circumscribed area of one of the major disciplines. For the foreseeable future, however, this would exacerbate the existing shortage of health care personnel in sparsely serviced areas. In addition, limited licensure would have to be adopted generally in North America; it would not be realistic to adopt it on a regional or national level.

An intriguing, although perhaps impractical, mechanism by which physicians might be motivated to strive for continuing professional competence would be a scheme of incentives. In our society, the most effective ones are financial. A study of the broad implications of this approach would be useful.

In some quarters, it is held that participation in continuing education programs must be compulsory and that relicensing must be dependent upon a practitioner's participation in such programs. It is further suggested that educational institutions conducting compulsory programs be charged with responsibility of certifying to the licensing or regulatory body that individual practitioners have compiled with the educational requirements. This might well be an ultimate goal, but it would have to be preceded by total university responsibility for the graduate phase of medical education.

Since continuing education is a new responsibility for the university, one might well ask what are the risks and what are the benefits to the university from, for example, a physician-in-residence program? As to risk, exercising responsibility for ensuring continuing competence would impose a heavy burden on the university and particularly on departments of continuing or postgraduate education. It is imperative that this new responsibility not interfere with undergraduate and graduate programs. Significant increases in staff, faculty, and in budgets will be necessary.

As to benefits, there appear to be at least three probable ones. Such a program would make a significant contribution to the quality of medical practice in affiliated communities, something that has only recently become of real concern. Secondly, the university could build a much needed new relationship with physicians, a relationship that is known to favorably influence the flow of patients to university hospitals and expedite regionalization of costly facilities and services. Finally, the physician-in-residence, the physician on sabbatical as it were, can enrich the teaching of the medical school by making the students aware of some aspects of the "real world" that may be overlooked by the faculty or outside their experience. The program would also foster the development of a more open-ended educational system and could hasten the introduction of the concept of recycling.

There are some other items, too, that deserve consideration. First is the impact of the intellectual challenge to the physician in practice who is responsible in part for the training of physicians' assistants and other health professionals. Second is the impact of the elimination of many diseases and the new thinking and practices this forces on the practicing physicians. Third is the impact of modern data storage—the accumulation of increased amounts of new and more sophisticated data on each patient and on healthy people as well, and the need to reeducate physicians to cope with this wealth of information. Fourth is the need for physical and financial planning if a scheme such as a physician-in-residence program is to be a successful component in the total health care delivery system.

In the long view, efforts to maintain professional competence must be supported by substantial changes in postgraduate training programs. These are necessary to ensure that new physicians will regard formal continuing education for themselves as a matter of course, not as a matter of choice. One proposal for experimentation in the postgraduate sphere is for the training of clinical scholars. It is worthy of more detailed description. Designed to fill the critical need for a counterpart to the physician-scientist, someone who will function intellectually and practically at the interface between scientific advance and clinical practice, these clinical scholars will be expert clinicians who are trained to be first-rate teachers.

Neither undergraduate nor graduate students are consistently exposed to critical analyses of the validity of diagnostic procedures, the consequences of particular types of therapy, the natural history of disease in treated and untreated states, or the long-term results of particular methods of treatment in given groups of patients. Furthermore, the design of clinical experiments, the problems of statistical analyses, and the understanding of the variables associated with human experimentation are not part of the body of knowledge that the average student takes with him when he has finished his formal training.

The scholarly skill of the clinical scholar will lie for example, in the following areas: educational principles and techniques as they apply particularly to medical and paramedical education; data collection and storage; computation techniques and statistical analyses as applied to the study of the natural history of diseases and clinical investigation; the design and interpretation of experiments; the development of techniques to study the efficacy of practice methods in the community; economic and social organization of medical care; and the principle of systems and other analytic techniques as applied to the organization and practice of physicians and paramedical personnel. In addition, some of these men and women may choose to develop special skills in administration, in government and politics, in urban renewal and problems of city design, in minority group problems and education, and in the history and philosophy of medicine and science.

This program would open up multiple career tracks coincidental with the changes occurring at the undergraduate level and in keeping with the aspirations of some of our best medical students and house staff. At the moment, they are discouraged by the absence of effective training programs. There are two critical areas where large numbers of clinical scholars are needed. The first is in our medical school faculties, for many of the problems that confront our profession today would be so easily solved at the source were this type of competence presently available. The second important role for these individuals would be as leaders in revitalized community hospitals.

Author's recommendations

1. The feasibility of recertification, relicensure, and the use of a scheme of incentives as a mechanism for motivating physicians to maintain a high level of professional competence should be exploited. Needed for the recertification process are individuals with expertise in evaluation and fiscal resources.

2. Technology in the audiovisual area should be further developed and employed in the continuing education of physicians. Wider use of the evolving patient data storage systems should be encouraged as a means for appropriate review of physician performance and as a stimulus to continuous self-renewal by physicians.

Coauthor's comments

Dr. Van der Kloot:

Taken as a whole the basic medical sciences have failed to contribute directly and effectively to the continued training of physicians. Probably there are two major reasons for this unhappy record: lack of practice and the unavailability of an appropriate forum.

Practice is essential for the development of any teacher; only by direct experience can an instructor come to understand the needs, interests, and the proper level of approach to the students. Extensive practice in teaching medical students is of amazingly little value when one is suddenly confronted with an audience of practicing physicians; the usual response is to take refuge in a detailed, precise exposition of scientific data. Too often the result is boredom and poor communication.

If plans are implemented to bring practicing physicians routinely back to medical centers for a reeducation period, then basic scientists will have a real chance to learn how to communicate effectively with this group. The results should be worth the inevitable initial frustrations and disappointments, but it will be a shame if the enterprise ends there. The really successful lectures and demonstrations should be recorded on video tape. In the next few years the ready availability of home video tape recorders will revolutionize continuing education. Physicians could subscribe to a service providing them with outstanding reviews of basic science along with the latest advances in clinical practice that could be viewed in their own homes and at their own convenience. Such a system could incorporate a telephone answering system to which the physicians could call in questions that could then be answered by mail.

But even if these developments take place, there is still a tremendous need for a periodical devoted to keeping physicians up-to-date with basic science and modern views of disease mechanisms. Today one of the most important communication devices in science is the *Scientific American,* which is largely responsible for keeping physicists aware of progress in biology and vice versa. This superb magazine is successful because of the excellent scientists selected as writers, the copy is thoroughly edited to ensure a proper level of approach and clarity of expression, and the illustrations are of the highest quality. A publication based on the same formula but devoted to advances in medical sciences would be a major contribution toward the continuing education of American physicians. I believe that one of the most substantial contributions a foundation could make would be to undertake the initial subsidies necessary to start the publication of such a magazine.

9. On creating a true continuum of medical education

Donald N. Medearis, Jr., M.D., and
Thomas D. Kinney, M.D.

The most important issue facing medical education is that of developing programs to meet not only today's but tomorrow's needs. To achieve this goal, the authors of this book are convinced that medical education must be decompartmentalized and redesigned as a true continuum extending from secondary school through college, medical school, hospital training, and postgraduate education. Medical and university education must be integrated so that new pathways will open to those seeking other than traditional types of medical careers. This chapter explores the possibilities for attaining an orderly system of medical education.

It would be satisfying to believe that the student who desires to become a physician could do so in an intelligently planned and well organized manner. This is not now the case. Our students' progress is not orderly nor has it been very intelligently planned. There is little continuity from one stage to another in our medical educational system. Consequently, valuable time is lost and much effort is expended needlessly.

A logical system would consider the future physician's education as a continuum beginning when the student makes his decision to study medicine and ending with his retirement. The various components of our educational system should be structured so that the student can advance from one to the next with the assurance that he will be challenged at each stage by new experiences pertinent to his career goals. In order to do this it will be necessary to evaluate the major changes that already have taken place in each component, pinpoint areas where further change is needed, identify factors that appear to be hampering the system, and devise effective methods to achieve continuity between all components.

Secondary school education

Everyone knows that significant additions have been made to our knowledge in all fields of science during the past thirty years. Our primary and secondary schools, aided by the National Science Foundation and various other learned societies, such as the American Institute of Biological Sciences, the American Institute of Physics and the American Chemical Society, have kept pace by developing courses of considerable rigor in science and mathematics. These courses have certain characteristics in common. They are intellectually demanding and require a much higher level of thought than those taught fifteen years ago. They are organized around major concepts, and they force the student to learn how to interpret information as it relates to these concepts and to apply this knowledge creatively. As a result, material that once constituted a rather standardized liberal college education is now familiar to many students before they enter the university. Most colleges and universities now encourage these better prepared students to enter with advanced standing, and have devised new curricular structures and learning experiences to satisfy their needs.

Ways must be found to guide promising high school students to institutions that will allow them to make the most of their academic achievements and abilities and will offer the best educational pathways to medical school. Otherwise, the student may find that he has entered a college which lacks the resources and faculty to provide an educational experience of sufficient rigor to prepare him for the demands of the modern medical curriculum. Students who attend such colleges are at a great disadvantage when they compete for admission to medical school and if admitted, often have great difficulty in performing on the same level as classmates.

Statistics for the year 1966 are a case in point. A total of 783 colleges and universities each provided at least one first-year medical student; less than half of them, or 335, provided 90 percent of the entering class; and only 3 percent, or twenty-five schools, provided 28 percent of medical school freshmen. This situation has been relatively constant throughout all the years for which data are available, and there is no evidence to indicate that it will change. It is hard to understand why a small institution with limited resources would try to maintain the expensive resources for the preparation of such a small number of successful premedical candidates. It would be fairer and more efficient for such colleges to direct the premedical students elsewhere. There is an obvious need for wiser and more informed counseling of prospective medical students. Acting along and with the Association of American Medical Colleges, the medical schools should make a vigorous and sustained effort to make secondary school counselors more cognizant about quality premedical schools.

Collegiate education

The quality of college education, especially in the sciences, has been enhanced by the upgrading of secondary school teaching. As a result, more and more premedical students are enrolled in advanced and unusual collegiate curricula and all premedical students are better educated than ever before.

Once in college, the student should be advised as to the various options for entering medical school and as to alternatives in health and related careers. There must be earlier and more active dissemination of information about courses, honors programs, and special programs in human biology which, in turn, might lead to early admission to medical school. This should occur during the first semester of the freshman year.

Content of the premedical curriculum. There is a great lack of unanimity regarding the body of knowledge a student should acquire in preparation for medical school. The pertinent literature is filled with pleas that the prospective medical student have a thorough grounding in the humanities. There are equally eloquent dissertations on his need for thorough grounding in the sciences. On the one hand, we are told that unless the student is versed in philosophy and the social sciences, he will not understand himself and the world in which he lives; and on the other, it is claimed that he cannot acquire a working knowledge of the science of medicine unless he has made a heavy investment of collegiate time in biology, physics, chemistry, and mathematics.

Consideration of these opposing pleas leads to the suspicion that there is no one way to approach the study of medicine. Most essential are the individual's development of proper habits of study and reading, of the ability to solve problems and of a desire for knowledge and understanding. If these traits are fostered, the student should be well suited to the study of medicine. That students entering medical school have widely divergent backgrounds should be applauded and not deplored.

Nevertheless, there are ways in which the premedical experience could be improved. One of the major drawbacks of present college curricula is the manner in which science teaching is compartmentalized. Compartmentalization is desirable during the development of a discipline when it brings together individuals working toward the expansion of knowledge in a particular subdivision of science. As the individual discipline grows, however, it tends to become detached from its parent source and to become an end in itself. Compartmentalization of science then becomes characterized in part by authority based upon specialized knowledge, and this authority becomes formalized with departmental status. Although helpful in the development of a field, the process of compartmentalization tends to produce isolation and reluctance on the part of its faculty to integrate its teaching with that of other disciplines. Such exclusiveness may serve the science major who wishes to confine himself to a single discipline, but it can seriously hinder the premedical student who needs to achieve a working knowledge of more than one branch of science.

Science teachers in the better colleges and universities, well aware of the dangers of compartmentalization, are experimenting with core courses in biology and integrated teaching of chemistry and physics. For example, the recognition of the unity of form and function in the cell is having far reaching consequences in collegiate courses in biology. Among other things, it has deemphasized the traditional dichotomy of plant versus animal, minimized descriptive biology, and substituted the study of key mechanisms of living systems, such as replication and homeostasis.

A logical extension of these newer approaches to the integration and teaching of science is the development of a coherent curriculum in human biology at the college level. This approach has been discussed in some detail by Dr. London in an earlier chapter. There are many advantages to be gained from such a curriculum not only for the student of medicine but for all students. Chief among them is the greater understanding of man and his place in the world. Such a curriculum could permit the student to bypass many of the basic sciences courses in medical school and begin his clinical studies sooner.

Some universities now offer undergraduate students the opportunity to take medical school basic science courses en route to the bachelor's degree. There are a number of advantages to such an arrangement. It provides another entry point into medical school after students have demonstrated their interest and competence in medical school course work. It provides the nonscience major and the educationally disadvantaged student with an opportunity to avoid the pressure of the first year of medical school by completing some of the basic science requirements in college. In medical schools where the curriculum is flexible enough it permits the student to complete medical school in a shorter period of time. It is conceivable that in the near future the only identifiable common experience for the students in some medical schools will be a year of prescribed rotation through certain clinical services, preferably with some selection alternatives.

The impact of these new approaches to science education has not yet been fully felt in the medical schools, but there is no doubt that it will profoundly affect their curricula as time goes on. Already there is a moderate amount of duplication in the content of college and medical school science courses. This trend will likely increase as the colleges upgrade their courses to meet the challenge of entering students with better science backgrounds.

Many college science courses already provide better preparation for medicine than their counterparts in the medical schools.

Medical schools must reassess the body of knowledge essential to a physician and determine how much of the new biology, chemistry, physics and mathematics is needed to practice medicine, to engage in medical research, and to deal with the socioeconomic problems of health care. Only the medical school faculty can determine the educational objectives for each component of the curriculum and these objectives must be consonant with societal needs and goals. These educational objectives should be expressed in terms of student behavior which can be measured. The three basic behavioral patterns upon which the student's progress through the components of the continuum would depend are: performance in objective tests of knowledge; ability to acquire, synthesize, and apply information in an appropriate test situation; and ability to solve problems in situations relevent to the educational objectives of the course or curriculum.

The medical schools also should determine how their basic science teaching should be altered in response to the better preparation of students. Better communication will be needed between faculties of the college and the medical school if there is to be more integration of the premedical and medical curricula. One starting point would be for each medical school faculty to initiate a joint conference with the university faculty to discuss overlapping course content and common goals. This might lead to mechanisms for further interchange.

It is always well in making changes to keep in mind the great variation in the backgrounds and educational experiences of students who desire to study medicine. The superior student who has reached a high level of achievement early in his scholastic career and who has made an early decision to study medicine ought to be allowed to enter medical school as soon as possible. Later entry should be possible for those students who have made their decision later and also for the students who acquire knowledge at a slower pace. While the early achievers might possibly enter medical school after two years of college, the slower ones should have the equally honorable option of entering after five or six years. Ideally, there would be multiple entry points from other health and science careers at appropriate levels and multiple exit points at varying levels of career differentiation.

Education in other health professions

The concept of a continuum should not be confined to the education of physicians alone. It is equally valid for all occupations and professions that relate to health. Flexibility of curricula to encourage individual programs leading to a wide variety of health careers should be the keynote of the system for the future. Such a continuum would require new patterns of give and take between the medical school and its parent university, between the university hospital and the surrounding community.

One of the great problems in the education of health professionals has been the great disparity between the quality and content of the education offered to medical students and that offered to those in the other health professions. Improving the quality of faculty and programs in the paramedical area and thus breaking down the educational barriers which hinder vertical and lateral mobility between the health professions would be a great aid in providing a common basic background for all health professionals. For example, parallel courses in science could be replaced by courses broad enough to serve more than one profession. If this alone was done it would minimize the time and effort required to shift from one career to another, and do much to eliminate the dead-end careers in the health profession.

Here again a case may be made for the teaching of human biology during the college years. Having access to this medical knowledge at the undergraduate level will improve mobility for the allied health students and will foster the development of new health careers in such fields as bioengineering, biomathematics, as well as others that require a knowledge and understanding of the human body.

Integration of medical school and university

The only effective way to develop a logical and well integrated educational continuum for physicians and health professionals is to have greater involvement by our universities at all levels of the educational experiences. Society depends upon the universities to anticipate the future, if for no other reason than that the universities have the responsibility of educating our youth for the future. In response to the public's increasing concern about all aspects of health care, the universities must help society anticipate its overall health programs for the future and prepare to meet them by educating health professionals who will have the needed knowledge and skills.

There should be greater coordination within the university of the many activities and programs that contribute increased understanding of the factors that influence human health. This will require imaginative new arrangements to permit and encourage the involvement of scholars and scientists in addition to those on the medical school faculty. Medical school courses should be available with appropriate restrictions to students in other professions and disciplines. Courses in other schools should be readily available to medical and graduate medical students. In order to make this possible, scheduling of medical school and university courses and curricula should be made compatible.

In addition to acquiring the knowledge and techniques of their profession, physicians must also learn to understand the health care system and the specialized occupational groups that make it function. They must also develop an informed and sensitive appreciation of patterns and their effects on health in their communities. Education in all of these areas is available in the university medical center, but it is offered to physicians only in bits and pieces. The problem is not to create new educational experiences but to realign those we have.

Those who will work together in the health professions should have the opportunity of learning together while in school. College courses in human biology should be open to students preparing for a wide diversity of careers including law as it pertains to medicine, health-care social work, physiotherapy, nursing, and research in human biological sciences. In graduate school, the university should provide opportunities for the nurse, the social worker, the physician's assistant and the physician to work together in situations approximating those they will encounter in the delivery of health care.

Graduate education—residency training

As pointed out in a previous chapter, the majority of medical schools in this country are making major revisions in their curricula. Most allow up to two years of elective studies. As a result, many medical students graduate with specialized and differentiated educations and the content and structure of residency programs must be modified accordingly. In particular, this means that the faculty of the university's medical school should accept responsibility for the graduate training programs for interns, residents and clinical fellows. When graduate medical education is no longer the sole prerogative of faculty oriented to individual departments or single areas of specialty practice, there will be an opportunity for experimentation.

It is unreasonable to expect universities to be innovative if they are forced to cope with a host of external accrediting agencies, boards, residency review committees, associations, and federal and state subdivisions, all pressing their viewpoints and surrounding their own regulatory areas with increasingly complex and repressive guidelines. For this reason, accreditation of all medical education should come under the scrutiny of one coordinate body whose function is to protect the public and maintain the standards of the profession.

These suggested changes will not come about easily but they can be accomplished if they are allowed to evolve in an orderly manner while the objectives are kept clearly in view. Since the new educational patterns must eventually become part of the universities, they should ideally originate there. It is important, therefore, to encourage the universities to participate actively and creatively in the education of health professionals. If the universities accept this responsibility, then a truly integrated system of education for physicians and all health professionals can be developed.

Summary

Medical education should be a continuous integrated learning experience stretching from college years through medical school, postgraduate hospital training and throughout the years of medical practice. Each stage should be a preparation for the next, but requirements for progression should be adaptable to individual motivation and needs.

This suggested continuum is not confined to the training of doctors of medicine but makes room for all the occupations that relate to health care. Flexibility to allow individual choice of studies leading to a wide variety of health careers would be the keynote of the system. It would require new patterns of give and take between the medical school and its parent university, the hospital, and the surrounding community, and would allow both vertical and lateral mobility through its curricula for both, with the aim of making the most economical and efficient use of university teaching facilities and of abolishing rigid course requirements that serve no really useful purpose. Continuity, flexibility, and individual choice of health careers would guide each student's course of study in college, in medical school, in postgraduate education, and in life. The aim of such an educational continuum would not be to inculcate large bodies of knowledge, but to teach the student to think, to solve problems, and to find and apply new information when necessary.

The university is the logical institution to exercise the responsibility for the education of health professionals as well as medical students. It should also take the lead in the planning, designing and operation of health care systems and in the creation of new knowledge essential to progress in health.

Author's recommendations

1. Medical education should be designed as a true continuum extending from secondary school through college, medical school, hospital train-

ing, and postgraduate education. The concept of a continuum should be extended to the education of all health professionals.

2. Both medical schools and the Association of American Medical Colleges should devise better systems for guiding students who want to study medicine.

3. Premedical college students should be advised during their freshman year about the new options for entering medical school and about college alternatives in health and related fields.

4. Medical schools should reexamine their requirements for admission in the light of upgrading of science courses in secondary schools and colleges.

5. Medical schools should make a greater effort to work with college faculties to bring about a greater degree of integration of premedical curricula.

6. Medical school faculties should take greater responsibility for improving the quality of the education of all health professionals.

7. Health professional education, and in particular the entirety of medical education from college through post-M.D. residency, should be the responsibility of the university.

Coauthor's comments

Dr. Stead:

Experience has shown me that medical students are willing to make a much greater commitment to the hard sciences and mathematics than are other health professionals. The attempt to mix medical students, nurses, and physicians' assistants in course work is generally unsuccessful and does not result in the development of teams which work together effectively. After all, doctors have dated nurses, courted nurses and married nurses with no effect on the professional behavior of doctors and nurses. One can more successfully mix these groups at the patient interface. The medical student will not learn introductory medicine, the methods of physical examination, electrocardiography, care of fractures, clinical pharmacology, and care of the patient with hypertension any faster than other persons with much less preparation in science. Mixing is intuitively tried early and, if this fails, it is never attempted again. Once more, we learn that observations are more useful than intuition. Team concepts are best learned at the doctor-patient interface, and here a team approach to patient care can be easily developed.

10. Family practice

No other section of this book has been discussed or debated as vigorously by the coauthors. There is some consensus on the problem and the need. In approaching the solution, however, there were two widely divergent and polarized points of view. Hence the chapter is presented in two sections.

In the first, Dr. Stead, with the assistance of Dr. E. Harvey Estes, Professor and Chairman of the Department of Community Health Sciences, Duke University Medical Center, has enunciated the multiple dimensions of the problem, some of the reasons for its existence, and society's need for a solution. Drs. Stead and Estes propose a solution that represents a radical departure from the current system of medical education with a separate admissions committee and a totally different curriculum than is used for the production of other physicians in the same academic medical center. They also suggest a separate mode of licensure.

In the second section, the other coauthors of this book propose alternate views regarding the mechanism of solution by providing bona fide opportunities within the existing framework of medical education to produce the providers of primary medical care. They also enunciate the liabilities to society in the first section.

Family practice: one view

Eugene A. Stead, Jr., M.D.

The Problem and Need

The authors of the various chapters of this volume are in general agreement when they discuss the problems of undergraduate medical education, the role of the university in graduate education, the development of residency programs, and the financing of medical education. Their ideas are less formal and their conclusions much more tentative when they discuss the problems of the physician in the delivery of health care to families.

Patients want to be able to pick up the telephone at any time of day or night and contact a doctor who can take care of their needs. They want to call the same number to obtain care for the child, the pregnant wife, or their aging parents. They want the doctor to be located at a geographically convenient place, with adequate parking. They want to know what the services will cost and they want a way to incorporate the expenses into their yearly budget. They want insurance or the government to cover the major portion of the expense.

Patients are not too concerned with the way doctors organize their practice to cover these few things that they believe are essential. They will accept solo practice or group practice in various forms. They do not have strong feelings about the use of paramedical personnel, nurse practitioners, physicians' assistants, or automated histories. They trust the doctor to keep his shop in order and to arrange his affairs so that they will obtain competent, efficient services.

The primary medical services desired by the public can be delivered by generalists working alone or in combination with other generalists; by generalists in combination with other specialists; or by internists, pediatricians, obstetricians, and gynecologists working alone or in groups. In the past, most generalists have worked alone or in groups where medical educators have felt that it is difficult to insure quality control, continuing education, and effective referral patterns. Many educators also believe that the consumer will eventually demand care by doctors who are at least as specialized as the present internist, pediatrician, and obstetrician-gynecologist. They believe that an increase in the output of internists, pediatricians and obstetricians and a change in the method of paying doctors will eventually force enough redistribution of doctors so that health services by these specialists will be readily available to all our citizens. This may be both the most expensive and least satisfactory way to deliver personal health services.

The authors of this section believe that the majority of the needs of an average family can be cared for by a generalist and that he can do this more efficiently and more cheaply than the more specialized internist and pediatrician. The internist in particular is trained to care for patients who are interested in making a major investment of time and money in health care. An internist does not practice internal medicine by the certificate on his wall. He cannot practice internal medicine, regardless of his training, unless he arranges his day so that he can give time and thoughtful consideration to the problems of each of his patients. The end result is a higher unit cost and less units of service per day. The generalist, by choice, sees a greater number of patients, does those things that can be done in a short time and refers to his specialist colleagues those problems that are more time-consuming for both the doctor and patient. He can lance a boil, remove fragments of glass from the eye, set a simple fracture of the wrist, determine if a chicken bone is stuck in the throat and attend a normal delivery more efficiently and more cheaply than a group of specialists.

The pediatrician and internist have another disadvantage in the practice of family medicine. They are oriented toward the care of the individual patient, and they may use up all the resources of the family in a hopeless struggle for the survival of a particular patient. A doctor caring for an entire family is less likely to use its total resources unwisely.

The authors of this section are not wise enough prophets to know how physician generalists will fit into the pattern of medical practice in the next fifty years. We believe they could be a very effective component of the health care chain composed of the nurse practitioner, the nurse specialist, the physician's assistant, the physician generalist, the internist, the obstetrician-gynecologist, the general surgeon, and the various subspecialists. We expect institutional forms to develop which can insure high quality of services and continued education for the health care professionals. We believe that emerging organizations responsible for the delivery of health services will be able to create more effective patterns for the delivery of personal medical services if they can add the generalist to their mix of professional manpower. To date, the states have licensed the doctor but have had no mechanism to insure that the doctor, once licensed, gives effective medical services or continues his professional education. Hospitals, through their boards of trustees and professional staffs, have frequently established standards for practice which are much higher than those required by the state licensing boards. We predict that the time will come when doctors are licensed to practice a portion but not all of medicine. These sections of practice will be made by both horizontal and vertical cuts. The horizontal cuts will be (1) general practice, (2) general surgery, (3) general internal medicine, (4) general pediatrics, and (5) general obstetrics and gynecology. The vertical cuts will include the more highly specialized and technically-oriented specialties. There will be mechanisms for peer review and mechanisms to require continuing medical education. Eventually, this type of differentiation between doctors will extend down into the medical school, and students will enter on their career paths before graduation. In time, some students will enter medical school to be generalists. Somewhere along the way, this fact will be recognized and this type of student will be educated and licensed as a generalist.

If the view is accepted that generalists are desirable, can the medical school and residency programs, as they are now structured, produce them? No one can as yet give a clear-cut, affirmative answer to our question. The output of our medical schools continues to move toward specialization. The number of generalists taking care of families continues to decline. There is as yet no clear evidence that the establishment of residency programs in family medicine will reverse this trend. We know that specialization is just beginning. The amount of knowledge continues to grow at an exponential rate while the brain, the processor of this knowledge, is being only slowly modified by genetics and environmental factors. The 25 percent of personal health services that cannot be handled by the generalist will require an ever expanding number and diversity of specialists. The question is not, "Can we discard the specialist?" Everyone agrees that is not feasible. The question is, "Can we discard the generalist?"

The family practitioner has several characteristics which differentiate him from other doctors. He is comfortable in giving personal health services to the children, the parents, and grandparents. He accumulates knowledge about his patients through a series of short contacts over a long period of time. He is able to deliver a large number of units of health services at a low unit cost and he is geographically located in a place that is easily accessible to his patients. The family practitioner extracts from the total pool of knowledge the parts that are useful in delivering high volume, low unit cost health services. He performs a specialized function in the community. Because of the excellence of their performance, the family practitioners are puzzled and annoyed when they are told they cannot be easily fitted into the medical school setting as faculty members.

When the family practitioner is practicing medicine in the community, he is the doctor specializing in a systems engineering approach to the delivery of health care. When he is in the medical center and not engaged in family practice, his unusual attributes disappear. We need to take the students to our professors of family practice and not move our family practitioners to the medical center.

The academic community is an organization dominated by specialists contributing their expertise to the general education of students who are going to be unlike themselves and to the specialized education of students who are going to be like themselves. The standing in the academic world of the specialists results from knowledge they have which is not equally shared by their colleagues in other fields. Family practitioners or primary physicians have to accumulate knowledge from a variety of specialists, but they have no specialized area of biomedical knowledge not known to other members of the academic community. The absence of an area of special knowledge makes it difficult to structure family medicine as a discipline within the university. Nursing has struggled with this problem without a successful solution; it has no area of expertise which is not known to other health professionals. We should not repeat in family practice programs the errors made in nursing. The leaders of the family practice movement appreciate their dilemma and are trying to buttress their academic standing by stressing the importance of the social sciences as a part of their educational program.

Since family practice does not have an area of specialized biomedical knowledge, the family practitioner takes additional work with specialists when he wants to increase his competence in any area of clinical medicine. This highlights what may be a fatal flaw in the residency programs for family practice. If the family practitioner goes to the specialist for additional training, why should not the student who wants to go into general practice also go to the same specialist for his graduate education? Why should not the medicine, pediatrics, obstetrics, gynecology, and psychiatry taught to the family practice resident have the same quality as that taught to the specialist?

Family practice programs set up outside medical centers suffer from lack of involvement of specialists in their educational programs. Family practice residency programs set up in medical centers are so artificial that they serve no real purpose. Most of their entering residents will eventually be drawn into other areas of specialization in the medical center.

One solution

One solution to the problem of establishing effective family programs would be to establish family practice programs as operating arms of broad-based departments of community health sciences. Community health sciences, drawing its members from medicine, pediatrics, psychiatry, gynecology, obstetrics, business administration, systems engineering, computer science, economics, sociology, and epidemiology, fits well into the present structure of universities and medical centers. Community-based professors of family practice could give this group an operating arm in the communities. A department structured in this manner could keep the medical school continually informed about the needs of the community and keep the community knowledgeable about the services available in the university.

Many of our colleagues believe that personal health services freely available and delivered by persons at least as specialized as our current pediatricians, internists, and obstetricians will greatly improve the quality of living and will result in a profound improvement in mortality and morbidity throughout the land. They are willing to invest whatever proportion of our resources are needed to give services of the quantity and quality which they believe to be desirable. They therefore decry as an attempt to give personal health services "on the cheap" the development of care which has a large unspecialized component.

We believe that there is much less gold to be mined by the delivery of personal health services by groups of specialists. Transportation, education, control of industrial pollution, population control, and adequate annual wages will have much more effect on the quality of living than will the development of an expensive and over-specialized system to deliver personal health services. Even if 75 percent of the services are given quickly, efficiently, and cheaply, the bill for the other 25 percent will be enormous. Any system of health care will cause some tragedies. The generalist will not refer some patients quickly enough. The specialist doing the work of the generalist will perhaps become bored and careless and let people die because he does not continue his role as a specialist under any system.

To restate the problem: can the medical schools produce generalists who are interested in providing high volume, low unit cost health services to the families of the nation? The answer *for the present* is probably no. What changes will have to be made to make the answer yes? The changes will have to be made (1) in the admissions policy, (2) in the curriculum in the medical schools, (3) in the faculty of the medical schools, and (4) in the graduate programs.

Changes in the admission policy, curriculum, and faculty of medical schools

Medical schools have a very restrictive admissions policy. They choose students who have received good grades in high school and college and they admit candidates from relatively few of the colleges. The object of the game is to admit students who can pass the basic science courses required in medical school. At first glance, the idea of admitting only students who are nearly certain to pass the medical school courses seems reasonable. On more careful examination, it may not seem so reasonable. The necessity of passing requires that these students come from colleges with professors quite like those in the basic science years of the medical school. It imposes a rather considerable homogeneity over the entire medical profession. The professors in the colleges preparing students for medical school are primarily interested in the fact that those students whom they recommend are accepted for medical school and do well in medical school. These referring college teachers are not interested in creating heterogeneity in the medical profession. Indeed, they have no leverage to do so because their students not fitting the medical school mold would be rejected.

The basic science faculties in the medical schools are not interested in admitting students who will do family practice. They are interested in students who will do well in their courses. The entire intake into medicine is thus controlled by persons who will never practice medicine. These admission policies produce excellent specialists and bioscientists. They do not produce many doctors who want to give primary medical care.

Primary medical care can be given by individual doctors who want to deliver care with their own hands or by managerial doctors who want to give primary care with a team of nondoctor helpers. The doctor delivering primary care with his own hands develops, by repetition, patterns of response to patients' problems which become as automatic as walking or running. He is thus able to give satisfactory high-volume, low-unit cost services with a minimum of intellectualization. He does not look on each patient as an opportunity for clinical research. He does what medicine has taught him to do and moves on to the next patient. He needs a well-run office, good support at the technical, secretarial, and nursing levels, and a place to hospitalize those patients who do not require an inordinate investment of time. The managerial doctor delivering primary care by the team approach can develop more time for thinking and planning. He has the support of a larger organization, and he is responsible for the continued development of this organization. The team delivers health service on the basis of repetitive, well-learned responses with a minimum of intellectualization. The doctor's intellectualization will be at the managerial interface rather than at the doctor-patient interface.

The medical schools need to admit three types of students: (1) the present varieties, (2) those interested in giving primary health care with their own hands, and (3) those interested in the managerial approach. Appropriate provisions need to be made to prevent the students in groups 2 and 3 from being flunked out of medical school by a faculty inappropriately using criteria designed to measure the capability of a different product. The students in groups 2 and 3 are not inferior students. They are students with different backgrounds and ambitions than those of the bioscience-oriented students.

The students in group 2 would be best selected from persons who have had some experience in the delivery of personal health services and whose applications were strongly supported by practicing doctors. The students in group 3 would be those who had shown interest and ability in the managerial sciences and who want to become involved in the delivery of health services. We propose that students in groups 2 and 3 should first receive a four-month introductory course in the delivery of health services to allow them to function as clinical clerks. After they have completed the two-year clinical clerkship, a medical school committee would decide the type and amounts of basic science and managerial science that each student needs to complete an M.D. degree and qualify him to be licensed as a generalist.

These proposed changes would give us the necessary breadth of input to allow medical schools to produce the widely differing kinds of doctors the health field needs. Our own observations convince us that we could produce very effective practitioners from each of the three groups. More but not all of group 1 should become specialists; more but not all of group 2 would give primary care with their own hands; more but not all of group 3 would practice medicine as the leaders of health teams incorporating modern methods of management.

The medical center would need to develop into a working laboratory for managerial scientists who have not normally in the past had space in the medical center. The departments of community health sciences would need faculty knowledgeable in business administration, economics, systems engineering, bioengineering, computer science, sociology, and the epidemiology of chronic illnesses. These new faculty members would teach medical students in group 3 and interact with graduate students from their own disciplines. They would form a nucleus of scholars which could act at the medical center–medical school interface on the one hand and at the medical school–practitioner interface on the other. If successful, these new faculty members would influence medical school curriculum and admissions policy and the patterns of medical care in the future.

Changes in graduate education

The graduate education of those students in groups 2 and 3 who want to practice family medicine should be under the direction of departments of community health sciences whose faculty would include physicians practicing family medicine in a variety of communities. A department of community health sciences needs financial support for residents to be trained in part by the traditional specialists and in part by practitioners in the community. The authors recognize the need for increasing experience in outpatient care in a model clinic and in the offices of community physicians. We also recognize the need for good specialty training.

After a year's experience in such disciplines as medicine, obstetrics and gynecology, pediatrics, or psychiatry, a family practice candidate could be profitably absorbed by another specialty service, since he would bring an expertise not normally present on the service. A man with a year's experience in obstetrics and gynecology who moves to medicine could function as the "office gynecologist" consultant to his colleagues. He could work on the medical service as long as needs be and not be a drain on the department of medicine budget since his financial support would be from his parent department.

Since family practice will be performed in the community by a variety of single doctors and also by groups of doctors, the type of competence to be acquired should be left to each candidate. All required rotations tend to be dull, and uninterested rotators can kill any service. This is especially true of surgical and obstetrical skills, which might or might not be needed in a given community setting.

During the period of graduate education in the medical center, the candidate for family practice should have experience in both managerial sciences and family practice in the community. The time for these experiences can be greatly augmented by giving him a good clinical support system. A nurse practitioner or physician's assistant would work with the family practice resident both in the medical center and in the community. Both should have access to a small computer reserved for their system of record keeping.

The family practitioner on the faculty would be paid for the time invested in teaching and for time devoted to effecting changes which would ultimately increase his ability to see more patients. The staff of the department of community health sciences would be a resource for the family practitioner interested in innovation.

In summary, we acknowledge the need for a doctor with more broadly-based skills who can function as a generalist and give primary care to the entire family. We accept the fact that the production of this product requires major changes in the composition of the medical faculty, the admissions and curriculum policies of the schools, and the programs of graduate education. We suggest that family practice departments staffed primarily by family practitioners will not be able to induce the changes in admissions policy, curriculum, faculty, and residency programs that must occur if generalists in large quantity are to be produced. Wider-based departments of community health sciences containing scholars capable of modifying both the medical school and the patterns of practice in the community are more likely to succeed. This model requires that these departments have a strong operating division of family practice. The family practitioners on the faculty would remain with their practices, but they would be well paid for a portion of their time devoted to the education of students and residents.

The following paragraphs describe a proposed training program for the preparation of tomorrow's generalist. The program assumes that there must be a different recruiting, a different training program, and a different postgraduate educational experience. It is assumed that this program would run parallel with the conventional curriculum of a well-established medical school and be the responsibility of the department of community health sciences.

Selection of students. Students will be chosen by a separate admissions committee who agree with the objectives of the program. Selection criteria will emphasize synthesizing rather than analytic capability, interest in primary practice as a career, experience in health care and experience with geographic areas or groups which are in particular need of health care (rural areas, areas with a high percentage of minority residents, etc.). There should be an attempt to widen the range of colleges whose graduates are admitted to medical schools.

Preliminary requirements. Before entering the first year, the student will be asked to spend several months working in the office of a generalist. His role will be similar to that of an informally-trained physician's assistant. The purpose is to acquaint him with the type of patient seen in primary care practice and the general characteristics of the services offered so that he will be able to contrast this with care offered in the hospital setting. For those with previous health care experience, this period of time might be spent in refresher courses at the undergraduate college level.

General characteristics of year one. The purpose of year one is to introduce the student to the words commonly used by the physician and to teach him how a physician thinks and works. It will be spent in the medical school and its hospital. The first four months will be largely didactic and taught by clinicians. The student will learn topographical anatomy and x-ray anatomy before he learns to dissect. He will meet the liver in the clinic and appreciate its function in health and disease before he meets the liver in the morbid anatomical laboratory. He will learn interviewing techniques and methods of physical and laboratory testing before he concerns himself with the sciences which have produced these methods of examination. He will learn facts about growth and development by observations of families. He will have enough epidemiology to be aware of the kinds of illness that are important in the patient population in the surrounding area. At the end of four months, he will begin his clinical clerkship. The practice of medicine will be interspersed with classroom work, laboratory work, and demonstrations by select members of the basic science faculty, chosen for their ability to relate their knowledge to the problems of the patient. The clinical instructor will attend the basic science lectures and laboratory exercises and relate the material presented to the problems presented by the patient.

Year two. There will be a continuation of the clinical clerkship in that the student will be assigned to hospital wards and work under clinical preceptors. The experience will differ from the clinical year of most medical schools in that patients will be assigned without regard to the nature of the admitting diagnosis. In fact, an attempt will be made to mix medical, pediatric, surgical, and other patients in order to simulate the mix of patients likely to be seen in the generalist's office. The objective of the year is to teach the student to achieve facility in the approach to the seriously ill patient and to learn responsibility for care of the seriously ill. Teaching rounds will be held on a daily basis, with the student and preceptor working together to derive maximum information from the attending specialists appropriate to the major problem. The base for this exercise will be in a community hospital rather than the university hospital.

Year three. This segment is designed to provide some exposure to management, records, the medical system, medical planning, and other components necessary for general practice. This material will be interspersed with patient experience in various office settings, with a large percentage of this experience being in general practice clinics. The objective of the clinical experience is to provide practical knowledge of the handling of relatively minor problems, achieving rapid turnover at a reasonable cost. This will be interdigitated with experience in relevant basic sciences such as gynecology, ear-nose-throat, and dermatology.

Year four. The student will spend this year as a responsible clerk in a family practice program in a community hospital. The activity and responsibility will be those usually associated with an internship year. The fact that the trainee has not yet received the M.D. degree can be met in one of several ways. The most interesting is to certify a student as a physician's assistant assigned to the chief of the service in the designated hospital. This could give him the benefit of some legal protection under legislation now under consideration in a number of states. It is hoped that these primary practice programs will afford both inpatient experience and outpatient experience in a primary care type clinic which should have its own record system, its own personnel, its own billing system, etc. The student might also profit by receiving a small percentage of the income produced in the clinic.

Postgraduate experience. Assuming that adequate inpatient experience in the care of seriously ill patients has been provided in earlier years, the student will spend his first post-M.D. year in the model family practice clinic and the offices of specially selected family practitioners, functioning as a member of these clinics for several months at a time. One rotation during this year should be in a university setting, such as the university health service where the trainee will receive exposure to survey techniques, computer-patient interaction, the use of physicians' assistants, and other newer techniques of potential future help in practice.

The second year of postgraduate training will be spent in specialty rotations in the medical center learning those parts of the particular specialties that will be most useful to him in his practice.

Licensing. The students graduating from these programs will have different aspirations and ambitions from those graduating from the specialty-oriented portions of the medical schools, and they should be licensed only for the practice of general or family medicine.

Author's recommendations

1. Between the physician's assistant and the physician specialists in internal medicine, pediatrics, obstetrics and gynecology, there exists a large area of health services that should be given by less specialized doctors known as primary care physicians who would provide high volume, low-unit-cost services.

2. To produce the required number of primary care physicians, medical schools must generate separate admissions committees to identify a different pool of students than is currently admitted.

3. Primary care physicians should follow a separate curriculum through medical school, take residency training largely in community hospitals and be licensed for the sole purpose of primary health care. A cross-over into specialization should be possible, but difficult.

An alternate view

William G. Anlyan, M.D., W. Gerald Austen, M.D., John C. Beck, M.D., William D. Bradford, M.D., Ray E. Brown, Martin Cherkasky, M.D., Lloyd C. Elam, M.D., Thomas D. Kinney, M.D., Irving M. London, M.D., Donald N. Medearis, Jr., M.D., William G. Van der Kloot, Ph.D.

Without doubt the need for primary care is great and as Dr. Stead has noted, the medical care system has not met, nor in its present form is it likely to be able to meet, the multiple demands and expectations of the American people. The continued fleshing out of our medical manpower resource by about two thousand foreign-trained physicians each year and our dependency upon large numbers of people with skills such as chiropractic, plus the unmistakable and repeatedly documented inadequacy in all parameters of health care for the poor, confirm his description of the state of affairs.

There are, however, alternative solutions to the problem that can be effected by appropriate changes in the existing continuum of medical education. We must be wary lest we be seduced by arguments that would ally us to standards easily and inexpensively achieved in place of a commitment to the goal of a single level of top quality health care for all Americans.

We must not try to meet the need for primary physicians by creating a medium-trained doctor who would be entrusted with great responsibilities, who would be better educated and more skilled than the physician's assistant but not as thoroughly prepared as the internist and pediatrician. Such an approach would ignore the lessons derived from the history of medical education over the past century. The suggestion that these primary physicians be educated essentially in an apprenticeship system is disquietingly reminiscent of the pre-Flexner period. It appears to be a recommendation born out of desperation, since it is a historical fact, and no accident, that for medicine the apprenticeship system failed in the early 1900s.

We should not allow ourselves to be lulled into a sense of nostalgia for the general practitioner of bygone days about whom there is a whole body of romantic remembrances. The truth of the matter is that when the general practitioner was the heart of medical practice there was very little for him to know and not really very much that he could do for sick people. The very notion of a generalist is antithetical to the existence of an ever-expanding base of medical knowledge and technology. As a result of the explosion in scientific information we have been able, increasingly since the 1940s, to base medical care on hard facts and the physician has become of greater value to the patient because of his knowledge, not because of his fatherly image.

All around us we find growing sophistication on the part of the layman about the quality of care and regardless of socioeconomic status, a keen awareness of the capabilities of modern medicine. People recognize full well that specialization means sharper skills and therefore greater potential for cure and for life and they want the best that medicine has to offer. They also want easy accessibility to those who can offer the best. Organized groups such as labor unions are no longer satisfied with the simple acquisition of medical services as a benefit for their members. They are now closely questioning the nature and level of that care and the quality of those who provide it.

And there is a steady decline of interest in family practice even among those physicians already established in it. At the University of Virginia School of Medicine, Drs. Ronald L. Crawford and Regina C. McCormack sent questionnaires to eighty-nine Virginia physicians who had left family practice. Of the seventy-three who responded, many complained that patients call on the generalist only for emergencies at night or on weekends, at other times and for most other problems going directly to specialists. About 29 percent reported some difficulty in securing hospital beds for patients. The cultural and recreational resources in the small communities where they lived were inadequate for 58 percent, and all complained that they had no private life. Without a discipline to call their own, lacking in status and acceptance among their peers and suffering professional and cultural isolation, they have moved toward specialization despite the fact that 25 percent were more than forty years old when they took this important step.

The position that most disease is self-limiting cannot lead us to the conclusion that primary care is simpler or that it does not require the doctor's time and intellectual capacity. The early decision in Russia to use feldschers in the rural areas was based on the erroneous notion that "simple" patients could go to primary care doctors and "complex" patients to specialists. All persons are complicated, and anyone's entry into the health care system should be via a highly trained physician who can determine when simple management is indicated and at what point more complex management is required. The primary care physician must be in fact the most skilled, the most thoughtful of all physicians. In many ways it is much more taxing and demanding to deal with the broad scope of health problems and concerns with which he is faced than to perform the most complex and fearsome surgery requiring enormous but more narrowly focused technical skills.

In this volume we are after all addressing ourselves to the education of physicians who will be practicing well into the twenty-first century, with the certainty that they will be forced to adapt themselves to continuing advances in scientific medicine, both in the ready assimilation of new knowledge and the capability of using it effectively. Can we now seriously consider limiting them to apprenticeship training, a static form of experience that provides little or no orientation to change and insufficient background within which to incorporate new knowledge?

The period of time specified by Dr. Stead for the training of this new variety of practitioner does not vary greatly from that required to educate the doctor. Dr. Stead stipulates that the candidates must be college graduates and then proposes that they spend four years in medical school followed by two years in a residency program of sorts. Yet, despite the investment those years represent both for society and the individual, we would not at their conclusion have medical professionals who by training, education, and motivation could meet any challenges that the future practice of medicine may offer. We would have instead practitioners limited to doing what they had been taught to do in the way they had been taught to do it. With more and more medical schools introducing the three-year curriculum and the internship being progressively eliminated, six years of medical school and residency will be sufficient to qualify a student for his boards in internal medicine. Under those circumstances, who would be willing to spend the same amount of time only to wind up with lesser status, less pay, and a profession lacking a clear discipline?

Only the multifaceted nature of the problem and the pressure of the needs could possibly find us at this time in history seriously contemplating the creation of a second-class doctor to serve a society well enough endowed with the resources, intellectual manpower, and money to provide medical care of the highest quality for all of its citizens. Since the American people have been inoculated with the virtues and desirability of quality health care and have shown their determination to seek it out whenever they can afford it, we can be quite certain that those with money or some special access to the system will continue to obtain the services of the highly specialized doctors leaving the poor and unsophisticated to the ministration of those less well trained. Do we really want to institutionalize for several more generations the inequities that now characterize our health care delivery system?

The solution to the critical shortage of medical manpower does not lie in the creation of a huge cadre of second-class doctors limited in skill and scope, but requires instead that we deal squarely with the need to increase greatly the number of highly skilled internists, pediatricians, and internist-pediatricians. According to the AMA, as of December 31, 1970 we had 58,000 general practitioners, 42,000 internists, and 18,000 pediatricians. Elsewhere in this volume, it has been recommended that the total number of physicians be quickly increased by at least 100,000. We should insist that this increase consist of first-class physicians so that every American can be assured of primary care of the highest quality. Let us broaden the selection of students to include those who have shown an interest in the social sciences and a lively concern for social problems. Let us rearrange the curriculum to educate students in psychology, history, anthropology, philosophy, and economics as well as in the basic underpinnings of medical science. Let us direct their entire training toward patient care but let us not fail to equip them also with a thorough knowledge of disease and the skills to diagnose it. Let us provide and encourage group practice arrangements, peer review, and the utilization of paraprofessionals to make maximum use of all our resources for efficient and economical patient care.

Primary medical care should have a firm base either in general internal medicine or general pediatrics or both. Obstetrics and minor surgery may be elective in the training programs depending on the interest of the trainee and his anticipated geographic and group practice setting. Primary care medical practice should be regarded as a specialty. The opportunity for subspecialization in emergency room care or in family practice should be available. The family practice subspecialty training program might include medical aspects of sociology, psychology, and public health as they pertain to family groups. Licensure should be in common with all other physicians.

With the advocacy elsewhere in this book of multiple entry points into the continuum of medical education, existing admissions committees should be broadened in composition and mission to insure that youngsters interested in primary medical care gain admission to medical school. With only 50 percent of applicants currently being admitted to medical school, there would seem to be ample reserve of talent within which to seek potential primary care specialists. It is unnecessary to look at new sources from colleges that have hitherto not produced any successful entrants to medical school in large measure due to the lack of adequate science programs.

Once the student is admitted, it is suggested that his tutor be selected from a pool of physicians interested in promoting primary medical care specialty programs. Weekly conferences on primary care during the required curriculum would assure a mechanism of reinforcement. The basic medical science elective period might include courses in the behavioral aspects of family and community care, epidemiology and public health. The clinical elective period should provide the opportunity to work in selected community hospitals and clinics with primary care specialists. The postdoctoral educational component should be located mainly in the affiliated community hospitals and clinics with backup resources of the university hospital. The training programs should be explicitly identified as primary medical care specialty programs linked to the academic medical center with committed involvement as needed by the clinical departments, especially medicine and pediatrics.

For continuing education also, the academic medical center and its affiliated community hospitals and clinics should provide multiple options for the primary care specialist and subspecialist similar to the opportunities currently afforded other specialists and subspecialists.

Authors' recommendations

1. The goal of top quality health care for all citizens should be met by primary care physicians who are highly skilled, thoughtful, and rigorously educated.

2. Primary health care is a specialty; physicians who practice it should have a firm base in internal medicine, pediatrics, or a combination of the two. Subspecialty areas of primary care such as emergency room care and family practice also exist. Licensure should be in common with all other physicians.

3. Medical faculties should make sure that students interested in primary health care are admitted to medical school and that their growth and development is promoted through flexible elective curricula.

4. Postdoctoral specialty training programs in primary health care should be based in affiliated community hospitals and linked to the academic medical center.

11. Manna from the physician's assistant program: a source of nourishment for medical educators

Eugene A. Stead, Jr., M.D.*

Consideration of the state of medical education reveals a remarkable sameness from school to school and from year to year. Most medical school faculties have had similar educational backgrounds because a relatively small group of schools sired most of those who have become the major decision-makers in our medical schools and because like begets like. Medical faculties are remarkably unsophisticated about the latent potentialities of working with different mixes of faculty, students and subjects, because all of their lives have been spent in recycling a single type of student through relatively fixed programs.

The arrangement of courses in the first two years of medical school and the creation of clinical electives in the third and fourth years has changed very little. Duke Medical School does now allow its students to become clinical clerks after eight and a half months of medical school, and it has also permitted some students to take third- or fourth-year elective courses before the fall quarter of their freshman year. These are the only significant changes in medical education which have occurred in the American system of medical education during the professional lifetime of the authors.

Medical school faculty engaged in the traditional training of medical students and graduate students for the biosciences have assumed only a minor role in the education of nurses and paramedical personnel. In 1964, the Duke Medical Center embarked on a new program that involved the clinical faculty of the medical school in the education of mature, employed high-school graduates who wanted to work with doctors in delivering personal health services at the community level. The students had previously worked in the health field and found satisfaction in their work. They were of good intelligence, had rapid rates of learning, and most of them were men who had served in the medical corps of one of the armed services.

* With D. Robert Howard, M.D., Director, Physician's Associate Program, and E. Harvey Estes, M.D., Professor and Chairman of the Department of Community Health Sciences, Duke University Medical Center.

The clinical faculty taught those persons, for whom we coined the now widely used title of "physician's assistant" * (or, for short, PA), how to interact with the patient and the doctor in such a way that more units of personal health services could be delivered by the doctor. The doctor–PA team was supported by nurses and conventional paramedical personnel. Two years of combined didactic and clinical work, with a high input of time from the clinical faculty, are required to train these assistants. The performance of our assistants has been excellent.

Persons with a high school education, a reasonable rate of learning, and a tolerance of the unavoidably irrational demands often made by sick people can learn to do well many of those things that the doctor does each day. Under the wing of the doctor, the PA can collect clinical data, including the history and physical examination, organize the material for use in diagnosis, and carry out any required therapeutic procedure which the doctor commonly uses. He can, of course, master any technical procedures which the doctor uses frequently. In fact, as a part of the doctor's team, he may perform so well that the patient cannot tell who is the doctor and who is the assistant.

The assistant is trained in the medicine of today. He can use the complicated technology worked out by medical scientists to help in the delivery of personal health services. He can use the tools that medical science has found to be helpful without necessarily understanding the theoretical basis for their usefulness. He can use established methods just as we use a radio without knowing much about the physical sciences that underlie its performance and design. For example, he can use the information obtained from measuring the blood pH, the bicarbonate concentration of the blood, and the pCO_2 without understanding the kinetics of hydrogen ions.

How then does the assistant differ from the doctor? Theoretically and ideally, the physician's education differs from that of the assistant's in the following manner:

1. The physician has a broad background of general knowledge which allows him to relate the activities of the healer to the broad aspects of society. He can appreciate the interplay between economic problems, environmental problems, governmental policy, and social change with matters concerning health. He can anticipate the kind of social problems that will result from exposing many of our young men to the military or establishing a specialized system of health care such as the Veterans Administration medical program.

2. The physician has the opportunity to learn a variety of symbolic

---

* Duke has since changed the title of the Physician's Assistant Program to the Physician's Associate Program.

languages which enable him to understand and use information about virtually any subject he wishes to master. He is thus freed from the necessity of memorizing large amounts of not-yet-needed knowledge since books and journals can give him this information as he needs it.

3. The physician has the opportunity to modify his brain and make it a more flexible instrument by using it to solve problems posed by those concerned with furthering knowledge in health fields. In the past, we have used the learning of bioscience as the primary means of modifying the student's nervous system. The uninitiated have thought that the content of these sciences was essential to the practice of medicine, but the more sophisticated have realized that the reward for such study was an overall increase in competence of the nervous system and was not directly related to the subject matter.

4. The doctor is taught the medicine of today by the apprentice technique, and the same technique is used in teaching the assistant. The method is effective in both instances. The apprentice experience of the doctor is interrupted by periods of study and nonapprentice learning experiences which can allow the doctor to become an independent thinker and worker. He learns languages and accumulates competences which are not directly related to the medicine of today but allow him to function effectively in the world of tomorrow. The education of the doctor is designed to prevent obsolescence in the face of changing social structures and a rapidly changing technology.

The reader will grasp the fact that the authors believe there is a great difference between the best-trained assistant and the best-trained doctor. We will also admit that the education of the doctor does not always achieve our theoretical ideal. It is probable that some schools and medical centers are training assistants and calling them doctors. How many of their graduates are independent thinkers? How many of them give leadership to their communities in matters of health and environment? How many concern themselves with intelligent adaptation to society? How many pursue a lifetime program of learning?

One question frequently asked is: should the physicians' assistants be an independent group, such as the nurses, or should they be an integral portion of the physician's health team? In the Duke program, we have opted for a high professional ceiling and have structured the PA as a dependent member of the doctor's health team. Most doctors have spent four years in college, four years in medical school, two years in the military service, and three or more years in graduate work before they enter practice. These doctors have had more years in the educational system than the young faculty who teach our children in college. We want the PA to profit from the years the doctor has spent in the educational system. As part of the physician's team, the PA can be taught more about illness and personal health services each day by his physician-employer-preceptor. After a few years of daily association with the doctor in the office, the hospital, the nursing home, and the homes of his patients, the PA will in all probability acquire a much greater competence than he had at the completion of his formal work in the medical center. Many lay persons have expressed the opinion that the PA should be licensed and be allowed to work independently. It is true that under the guidance and continued instruction from a doctor, the PA can carry out most of the functions of the doctor, but the doctor insures the quality control and the continuing education. If the PA were licensed independently, the functions he could perform would be severely limited by the terms of the license. He would have gained independence from the doctor, but he would not be very useful in the delivery of personal health services.

The physician's assistant must have a way to evolve from his dependent but effective position into one of independence. To accomplish this, the profession and the medical school must give due credit for the knowledge and skills learned as an assistant by making it possible for a properly qualified PA to go through medical school in less than the usual amount of time. Broadly-trained assistants who worked closely with physicians in family practice would not need to take most of the work commonly given in the third and fourth years of medical school, and many such assistants would also possess the skills usually developed by the doctor during his internship.

An assistant can be trained very broadly or very narrowly. The narrowly-trained assistant may become much more skilled in this area than 99 percent of the doctors in practice. His education can be given in three months to a year. The difficulty is that in most instances the narrowly-trained assistant will have a good many hours a day when he is not used optimally. The cost of operation skyrockets as personnel are not optimally employed. It takes longer to train a more general assistant, but if he can perform in the home or train others in the home to perform some of the functions normally assigned in the hospital setting to nurses, physiotherapists, dietitians, and laboratory technicians, costs can be reduced.

We have not written a job description for our assistants. We have given them a broad experience in the delivery of personal health services by having them work closely with doctors engaged simultaneously in practice and education. Doctors have the educational background to do many things but in actual practice each doctor recycles each day only a small fraction of those total activities once learned by all doctors. A broadly-trained assistant can easily adapt to the practice of any doctor, but it would be impossible to write a meaningful job description that would cover all the

activities which could be usefully performed by the assistant under direction of any doctor.

The incorporation of the PA as an integral portion of the physician's
health team will work if the medical school trains its medical students to
assume a broader managerial role and thus precludes the necessity of the
physician and the PA being in close geographic proximity. The assistant
does not have to be in the same room, or even in the same town, if modern
techniques of communication are used and if the quality of the service
rendered is the responsibility of the doctor.

Educators have long discussed the desirability of identifying areas in
which the education of the physician could be effectively combined with
the education of other members of the health team. Most such experiments
have been conducted during the period of preclinical training. In general,
they have failed, because health care learners other than the doctor have
not been willing to make the same heavy commitment to the learning of
biological science that is required of the future physician. We have had, on
the other hand, no difficulty in combining the assistant's education with
that of the medical student at the clinical interface. The assistant learns
history taking, physical diagnosis, emergency care of acutely ill patients,
electrocardiography, clinical pharmacology, diagnostic and therapeutic procedures as easily as does the medical student. In these areas, learning is
immediately translated into activity. One is not learning simply for the joy
of learning: one is learning so that he can work more effectively with
patients. Medical students, interns, and residents in the Duke Medical
Center have the opportunity to watch the physician-PA team at work.
The doctors in residency training participate in the training of the PA. The
PA will be used most effectively by those who have grown up with the
program and are not afraid of the PA's replacing the doctor.

Appreciation that the clinical material commonly learned in medical
school can be effectively taught to motivated high school graduates who
derive satisfaction from the delivery of personal health services and who
have a reasonably rapid rate of learning, opens up the health field to rural
and minority groups. No progress can be expected in this area when it takes
eleven years from the first day of college until the first day of practice. One
of two things happens at present. Commonly, the person from the rural
area or minority group just never tries to enter the system. The culture in
which he has developed does not equip him to plan for an eleven-year
period between starting a program and reaping the rewards of his efforts.
If by chance he does enter the race, he spends eleven years working with
people who are alien to his culture. In order to survive, he becomes more
and more like his classmates. By the time he enters practice, he has no

desire to return to the culture of his origin. We have seen this same phenomenon happen many times when students from Asia, Africa, and South America spend their college, medical school, and graduate years in the United States. They have excellent preparation for living in middle-class America, but do not thrive when they return home.

The assistant can be engaged in full-time work within two years. Under the direction and in collaboration with his doctor, he can continue to learn and grow professionally. The assistant then begins to see himself in a different light. When he discovers that he can work effectively with the doctor and is assuming an important role in his community, he will think in terms of making a greater commitment to education. A team of two assistants helping a doctor would allow each assistant to have six months of education per year in the medical center. Under such an arrangement, an assistant could move toward an M.D. degree without leaving his community base.

Many of our PA's want to have a college degree with a major in the clinical sciences. As presently carried out, the clinical education can precede two years of college work, can be interspersed between two years of college, or can follow two years in college. This flexibility has proven invaluable in recruiting students from rural and minority groups.

Medical schools could profit by similar flexibility. Some of the traditional college courses could be taken during medical school, and some of the traditional medical school courses could be taken during the college years. If the clinical experiences were given earlier, medical students could gain both money and experience by working as physicians' assistants with the family doctor.

The education of the assistant has raised certain questions about our medical schools' admission policies. The PA allows more flexibility in the construction of health care delivery systems. Within the next few years we will have some machine components ready for field testing. These new man-machine systems are going to require more managerial talent than we now have in medical schools. We need medical students who are gifted in economics, information sciences, systems engineering, business management, and certain aspects of sociology. We cannot bring gifted students from those fields into medicine if we require them to spend two years memorizing bioscience in order to become an M.D. We need to broaden our faculty so that these other disciplines can be used to educate medical students. The amount of bioscience needed to practice medicine can be taught to these students by clinicians as a part of the apprentice system of learning. They will practice as good medicine as those taught on a bioscience base. Their research interests would be in the fields of their original interest: namely, information sciences, engineering, business management, et cetera.

The change in admissions policy would need to be accompanied by a change in promotion policy, so that a single department could no longer bar a candidate from obtaining his M.D. degree. A department of biochemistry, physiology, or medicine cannot by itself determine whether a given person will make a satisfactory doctor. The functions of doctors today are too varied and the amount of postgraduate training too extensive to make the old promotion policies desirable.

The physician's assistant program at Duke has placed great weight on letters of recommendation from doctors who have worked with the prospective student. Medical student admission committees might profit by encouraging prospective students to gain experience in the health field by working with doctors. We know our medical students are bright, but we have no way to know whether they care for people.

The implementation of the education of the PA is the first step in the development by the Duke Medical Center of a clinical support system for its medical school graduates. In the past, we were content to graduate doctors and nurses and let them make their way in the community without any support from the Medical Center other than our programs for continuing education. We did not concern ourselves with a systems engineering approach in which we assumed responsibility for the development of all the men and machine components necessary to give effective health services to all segments of our society. The education of our nurses was not coordinated with the education of our doctors. The systems of education were so separate that no credit in medical school was ever given for any experience gained by a nurse.

It has been interesting to watch this attitude change. The clinical faculty of the medical school has accepted the fact that it is responsible for the entire system—not just the doctor. The faculty is willing to educate the PA and to allow undergraduate nurses to take elective courses in the medical school and to give them credit for this work if they wish to become M.D.'s. The Medical Center is making undergraduate degree programs available to its health workers. The Medical Center, in conjunction with the rest of the university, is developing programs in computer science and bioengineering which will allow new ventures in systems for health services.

In planning for medical education of the future, it is essential to consider the entire scope of the educational responsibilities of the medical school. All too often, programs of medical education designed by medical educators will recycle the past. They will focus entirely on the doctor. They will not give the doctor a support system that will allow him to function effectively in the delivery of health care to our society. We need more medical schools committed to the concept that they will produce all the component parts which are necessary to make the health care delivery system work.

Summary

1. Persons with a high school education, a reasonable rate of learning, and a tolerance of the unavoidably irrational demands often made by sick people can learn to do well those things which the doctor does each day. Under the wing of the doctor, such a physician's assistant can collect clinical data, including the history and physical examination, organize the material in a way which allows its use in diagnosis, and carry out any required therapeutic procedure which the doctor commonly uses. He can, of course, master any technical procedure which the doctor uses frequently. In fact, as a part of the doctor's team, he performs so well that the patient cannot tell who is the assistant.

2. The physician's assistant must have a way to evolve from his dependent but effective position into one of independence. To accomplish this, the profession and the medical school must give due credit for the knowledge and skills learned as an assistant by shortening the way through medical school for a properly qualified PA. Broadly-trained assistants who worked closely with physicians in family practice would not need to take most of the work commonly given in the third and fourth years of medical school, and many such assistants would possess the skills usually developed by the doctor during his internship.

3. The development of clinical support systems based on a permanent team of trained assistants rather than on the intern-resident educational model will allow medical centers and community hospitals for the first time to separate their service needs from their educational responsibilities. Cardiovascular surgeons made cardiologists honest. Good clinical support systems can allow educators to be honest. More units of service can be given by a team which consists entirely of trained manpower than can be given by a team which is giving service as a means of converting green manpower into trained manpower. The service demands of the university and the community hospital which are in excess of their teaching needs can be met more cheaply and effectively by the development of clinical support systems.

4. This is the only chapter in this book which considers the entire scope of the educational responsibilities of the medical school. Herein lies our problem. Programs of medical education designed by medical educators

will recycle the past. They will focus entirely on the doctor. They will not give the doctor a support system that will allow him to function effectively in the delivery of health care to our society. We need more medical schools committed to the concept that they will produce all the component parts which are necessary to make the health care delivery system work.

Author's recommendation

It is recommended that medical schools and their associated medical centers assume responsibility for producing all of the human elements necessary to deliver personal health services.

Coauthors' comments

Dr. Cherkasky:

It is hardly open to question that if in the various care programs, both those that include institutionalization and those which provide ambulatory care, we were to eliminate any element of education and focus solely on service, several things would happen. The diagnosis would be arrived at more quickly, the use of x-ray, laboratory, and other similar supports would be curtailed and definitive therapy would be applied more promptly. Therefore, patients would have shorter periods of hospitalization and the cost would be less. If this is the case, then why should any of our great hospitals carry on educational activities? Part of the answer lies in the undisputed fact that the existence of educational programs and the presence of questioning young people are, in themselves, an important stimulus to quality. Additionally, good professional people look for the opportunity to teach and find great joy in it. I am concerned that if the educational aspect were to be eliminated, there would not only be inevitable deterioration in quality of care but also that the very best people would lose their enthusiasm and drift off elsewhere. The most important single question raised is how do we educate a new generation of physicians and other health workers? I must say that I know of no way to teach a doctor except to let him doctor under supervision. When education begins to affect the economy and efficiency of service, for which third parties explicitly pay, they and their constituents complain. Actually, it does seem quite unjust that the hospitalized patient should carry the burden of an educational program that has value not to him alone but to the whole society as well. However, if we are to have future generations of highly skilled physicians caring for patients—and no new health worker I have seen or heard described leads me to conclude that medical care and practice in this country will be based on any other professional than the physician—then, in many institutions and especially in the best institutions, this admixture of care and education will have to continue. To resolve the problem, support of the educational aspects should be drawn from some more suitable source than payment by patients for services, and it is really not too difficult to make judgments about how much of a house officer's time fits into each category. The inefficiencies and longer hospitalization which are side effects of the learning process must be borne because they ultimately render the doctor of great value to the society. In my view, this is so whether or not new kinds of health workers assume some of the tasks which doctors have thus far performed.

Dr. Medearis:

Dr. Stead has proposed and developed a demonstrably effective program, that of the physician's assistant. There is another program which has equal if not greater effectiveness, one which involves the role of the nurse, the only professional other than the doctor who, on a twenty-four-hour-day, seven-day week basis, provides medical care. If utilized widely by our universities and their schools of medicine and nursing this program would provide many more qualified, baccalaureate-educated health professionals in a much shorter time and at less cost than Dr. Stead's program. Such programs as developed by Silver and Kempe at Colorado have demonstrated that the nurse can act effectively as a pediatric nurse practitioner in the pediatrician's office, and can effectively meet the need for another pediatrician in a group of pediatricians when one of them leaves. There is no doubt that one of the reasons she can act so effectively in the latter role is because a significant percentage of what the pediatrician does in his office is a professional activity, but one which can be performed effectively by less well-educated and trained individuals. (An educationally important corollary of this is that the pediatrician must become even more effectively educated and trained as the human biologist and student of abberations of normal developmental human biology). There is no reason why nurse practitioners, appropriately educated, would not be effective also in assisting the internist, the psychiatrist or the family care specialists.

There is, then, a demonstrably effective alternative to the education and training of health professionals to assist physicians that is quite different from that proposed by Dr. Stead. The education and training of the nurse provide a very meaningful base upon which to develop a professional fully qualified to be a physician's assistant as defined by the NAS report. Many such individuals could replace the physician in the delivery of medical care.

I believe that the physician's assistant should have a college education; it is invaluable in understanding the whole of society's affairs in which the physician's assistant must work. If nurses' aides and ward attendants could then be used to provide many of the services now provided by nurses, and if those nurses who were qualified could receive additional education and training, this process might provide very much more rapidly and very much more effectively than any other the number of health professionals needed in this country. To do so would require an effective liason between schools of nursing and schools of medicine. Some university nursing education already includes more specialists programs, the basic content of which in a number of instances could be easily adapted to that of the physician's assistant. Those universities with both schools of nursing and schools of medicine should develop programs housed within schools of nursing but participated in by schools of medicine. Their purpose would be to educate nurse practitioners; this should be a high-priority federally-funded program.

This program would have the following advantages: first, it would be based on a baccalaureate education; second, it would be housed in university schools of the health professions, medicine and nursing, which have an already demonstrated capability; third, the product of such programs would not require the change of licensure laws in most of the states of this country; fourth, it would capitalize on a demonstrably, remarkably effective working relationship between two health professionals who are already educated and trained to work effectively together, the doctor and the nurse.

I want to turn to another facet of this matter of the professionals for delivery of health care in the future. It cannot be too strongly emphasized that Dr. Stead's eminently reasonable and productive approach through the use of physicians' assistants is but one approach and one aspect of this matter. Although it might seem there is a clear overlapping of interests and capabilities between the physician and the physician's assistant, this, of course, is not the case. Physicians' assistants have been educated and trained in circumstances that leave no doubt whatsoever as to who was boss. Thus, any conflict between the professional and the paraprofessional as to who had the authority was resolved by edict uttered by the doctor. This is probably as it should be, but it is not as it will be in some other similar situations in which doctors and other professionals in health care delivery will interact. It is well for us to anticipate that with the increasing move toward professionalism, equality and autonomy on the part of the many and diverse elements which comprise the professionals and paraprofessionals who will deliver health care, there will occur a blurring of the margins of the roles they play. Conflict and stress will accompany this blurring. It will be felt least where the role of one professional is well defined and clearly supersedes and transcends that of another. Such a situation obtains between the cardiovascular surgeon and the "scrub" nurse. However, in the relationship between a psychiatrist delivering primary care in psychiatry and a psychiatric nurse therapist or a psychiatric social worker there will be conflict and stress because of the similarity of skills and activities. When there is excessive conflict, one might assume that the roles are really the same and that one or another of these professionals should withdraw either from that field or from that situation. In that instance, the more highly qualified should withdraw to do more demanding things, providing that standards of care have been developed to measure the performance of the less educated / qualified individual.

This approach will not solve the general problem; but understanding it will help. We must find alternatives to the sequence which now seems inevitable: increase in knowledge, information and technology, specialization, associations, separate licensure, separate bargaining, disintegrated programs in education and care, and irresolvable conflict which prevents the solution of societal problems.

12. Financing medical education

Ray E. Brown*

The health care delivery system is by all odds one of the most discussed components of contemporary American life. An uncountable number of national, regional, and local studies on this subject have produced their equivalent in generally thoughtful and statistically documented reports. Despite this tidal wave of findings and recommendations, things seem to get worse rather than better, and the cry of crisis grows louder. This does not mean that the studies and reports have had no effect. Their effects have been many and gigantic. Vast federal and state programs for financing patient care have been established and sizeable financial support has developed for research and demonstration in patterns of health care delivery. It does mean, however, that their effects have been regressive in that they fueled up demand without increasing supply.

Current problems in financing medical education

While the findings and recommendations of the many reports have been highly varied, and sometimes extremely divergent, they all agree on one thing—the crippling shortage of health manpower and the centrality of the physician shortage to the health care problem of the nation. No responsible policy maker can fault the reports for failing to call attention to the bottleneck that health manpower creates in the health care system and the crucial place that the physican shortage holds in this bottleneck. Despite this barrage of evidence and exhortations about the need for more physicians, the nation has not taken the obvious step necessary to produce them by giving medical education a high priority in the expenditure of its resources.

* While the author is solely responsible for the contents of this paper, much credit for both its substance and orientation belongs to the following individuals who met as a group with the author for a day's discussion of the subject: William D. Bradford, M.D., Duke University; Leonard D. Fenninger, M.D., National Institutes of Health; Matthew F. McNulty, Jr., Georgetown University; Joseph S. Murtaugh, Association of American Medical Colleges; C. H. William Ruhe, M.D., American Medical Association; James R. Turner, Children's Hospital Medical Center, Cincinnati; and Joseph A. Wells, M.D., Loyola University.

This is not to say that no official attention has been paid to the need for more physicians. "More physicians" has become the battle cry of federal and state legislators and is the condition they attach to any increased support for medical education. There is a generous willingness to provide inadequate support for added enrollment out of the already inadequate support available for existing enrollments. Because of their deep social concern over the need for more physicians and the financial problems that plague them, medical schools are expanding themselves into deeper financial distress and into academic mediocrity. Even this process of trading academic excellence and scientific progress for numbers is not sufficient, however, to meet the growing demand for physicians nor the growing aspirations of American students of all economic and cultural groups to be physicians.

A host of different studies and estimates pointing to a continuing shortage of physicians is reflected in *Manpower for Health—National Needs and Federal Programs,* a July 1969 report by a staff task force for health manpower of HEW. After reviewing existing enrollments, anticipated new medical schools, and expansion of existing ones, the report concludes that "even with a substantial increase in medical school enrollment during the next few years, the outlook is for a continued shortage of physicians. Unless there is a major social commitment to expansion of medical education, the increase in physician supply of the next decade probably will do little more than keep pace with population growth" (1).

Population growth is only one of the several major forces affecting the increasing demand for physicians. Of equal or greater influence are new health care financing programs, rapidly rising levels of personal income, new medical procedures, new definitions of illness and more emphasis on out-of-hospital and preventive care. Pressures on supply are also increasing as the need multiplies for more nonpracticing physicians, as physicians demand a shorter work week and shorter work life, and as the rate of importation of foreign physicians starts to decelerate. Some gains in supply are being anticipated from reorganization of medical practice and use of substitute personnel and electronic devices for physicians. It is difficult to see, however, any great impact of such worthy measures on physician demand. Beyond the computer and the battery of substitute personnel there remains the patient to whom all of these advances are of little satisfaction and value unless he gets his time with the doctor.

To pick a number for purposes of discussion, one could credibly use the estimate of the December 1968 Special Report of the Carnegie Commission on Higher Education that "spaces for about 75 percent more medical students will be required by 1976–77—above the spaces available in 1966" (2). This would mean about 16,000 first year places required by the fall of 1976 and a total enrollment of about 59,000. In 1971, there were about 11,000 medical school freshmen in a total enrollment of about 38,000.

Talking about demand *for* doctors tells only one side of the story when evaluating training opportunities. It may well be that the strongest pressures for expansion of medical schools in the future will come from the demand *to be* doctors. The notion is growing that a qualified person has a right to be a doctor just as much as a right to see a doctor. Actually, this idea has prevailed in all other professions throughout the history of this country. Only in medicine has need been used as the criterion for the number of training opportunities. Recognition of the right of particular ethnic and racial groups to study medicine was the basis for the establishment of some of our existing medical schools. The same recognition is now stimulating special efforts to increase the admission of students from minority and low-income groups. If the criterion of opportunity is used, the picture is clear and the figures are simple. For the 1969–70 first year class, there were 24,465 applicants for approximately 10,500 places, or 2.3 applicants for every place, and it is generally agreed that these applicants were fully qualified. The number of qualified applicants is expected to increase annually due to the rapidly increasing number of high school and college graduates, to the rising aspirations of students and their families for professional careers, and to the steadily increasing implementation of a social commitment to remove economic, racial, and sexual barriers to those aspirations. Indeed, there is evidence that the supply of applicants is self-fueling. Historically, the ratio of applicants to acceptances increases with an increase in acceptances and decreases with a decrease in acceptances. This correlation appears to reflect expectations rather than aspirations.

The health care system is plagued by manpower shortages at all levels, and some of these represent very serious difficulties in recruitment for training and in retention after training. Most classifications are low in status, low in pay, and low in career horizons with no career ladder available on which to climb. The problems of the physician shortage are quite simple in comparison. There is no significant difficulty in student recruitment and retention. The physician is at the top of the medical totem pole in every respect. There is only one real obstacle to ending the physician shortage: that is the difficulty of financing medical education.

There are, of course, problems in the medical school of program design, content, and duration. These have always existed and always will. They are currently acute because of the failure to confront them and correct them over the years. They can be handled and are being handled by the medical schools, however. The only crucial aspect of those problems is the possibility of overkill under the great weight of current social, economic, and political pressures for change in medical education. Medical education must change but it must not in the process, because of financial distress, short-change the potentials for the health of the American people. Like all education, medical education deals in futures, and the medical education of today is shaping the medical care of two and three decades from now.

Medical education requires facilities, faculty, and students, and all three in sufficient numbers are no further away than the right number of dollar bills. It is clear that the prospective students are waiting in the wings and the potential faculty are within call. During the sixties when the number of fulltime faculty, both basic science and clinical, doubled, the percentage of unfilled faculty positions ran steadily between 6 and 7 percent. This is a record that any other industry would be ecstatic about. One cannot fault the quality of the faculty members recruited either. To do so is simply to fault the medical education process itself. Medical schools have had first choice of the cream of their products. While faculty search committees may grumble about the competition, the competition is largely between medical schools for the best. Actually, the faculty vacancies that do exist are mainly the result of the deliberate and demanding process through which medical faculty appointments are made. The rapid upgrading of both salaries and supporting resources made possible by escalating sponsored research during the past decade has helped to attract excellence to medical school faculties. Any deterioration in available resources would, of course, handicap faculty recruitment in the future. The quantity and quality of future medical school faculty will depend on the finances available for the support of the tangible and intangible assets that attract and nurture first-rate medical scientists and teachers.

As to medical education facilities, dollars are the only bottleneck. Facilities dollars represent a much greater bottleneck than is recognized by those who control the flow of funds to medical education, both public and private. The hostilities toward "brick and mortar" support exhibited by foundations and many well-meaning individual donors, plus the reluctance of federal and state appropriating agencies to face up to the capital needs of medical education, have resulted in rapidly obsolescing and very inadequate medical education facilities in this country. The failure to recognize plant depreciation and to fund it has forced medical education to cannibalize its capital structure for support of its operating programs. It is becoming quite obvious that operating programs are increasingly dependent upon facilities and that much greater attention must be paid to plant needs and plant utilization in the future.

If the controlling obstacle to an appropriate increase in the number of physicians is dollars, a simple question emerges, "Why haven't the dollars been provided?" The answer is not as simple as the question and involves a number of factors, some of which have plagued this country's financing of medical education throughout its history. Before examining those factors, it should be understood that the most urgent financial problem confronting medical education is not the financing of increased enrollment but rather the adequate financing of current enrollment. With most of the privately supported medical schools, it is a matter of survival itself. No less than a dozen privately supported medical schools were forced into state operation or state support status during the past decade. The financial plight of all medical schools can only worsen if they are tempted into taking the bait of augmentation funds on top of already shaky budget structures.

Underlying the failure to provide adequate financial support in general to medical education, there is some skepticism as to the real urgency for financing increased enrollment. Perhaps most important is the view of a few respected health field leaders that our problems are not caused by a shortage of physicians but by our failure to utilize effectively those we already have. These spokesmen argue for more efficient organizational patterns for the health care delivery system, the use of substitute personnel for certain aspects of the physician's present functions, and greater orientation toward health maintenance and prevention of disease. As laudable as any of these methods might be and as capable as all segments of the health field might be to implement them, it is naive to predicate future physician manpower supply on these solutions only. All would likely increase accessibility and with it demand for physician's services. None, where implemented, has resulted in significantly increased physician productivity or in a significantly decreased demand for physician services.

A second element of doubt is the belief that some form of curricular magic could make room for more students within the existing budget and facilities. It is true that a number of important innovations are altering the content, length, and sites of medical training. The influence of these changes on the cost of medical schools, however, will not go far toward supporting the necessary increase in enrollment. Most of the functions for which the medical school is held accountable today will not be affected by such curriculum changes. Furthermore, much of the curricular change applies to the period beyond the M.D. degree which is largely beyond the budget of the medical school. While some of the innovations permit better utilization of facilities, they may actually decrease the efficiency and productivity of the faculty.

A third factor in the failure to provide necessary funds for increasing the supply of physicians has to do with the success of medicine itself. Since World War II, the public and the politicians have been inured to gloomy and scholarly predictions of health care crises expected to result from the physician shortage. None of these dire consequences has come to pass. This was largely due, of course, to the incredible victories medicine has scored against the germ-related diseases. Now that prospects no longer exist for medical bargains of this type, future medical advances will be marked by both their physician-intensity and long-term nature. Actually, all major physician manpower studies since World War II have underestimated both need and supply. Beginning with the Bayne-Jones report, the projected needs for physicians have been surpassed in each time period.

More important than the failure to finance increases in physician supply have been the conditions that have plagued the financing of medical education in general. They must be widely understood and corrected if medical education is to be spared a threadbare existence and a sharp deterioration in the high quality made possible in recent years by the windfall of research funds. Research support has now leveled off while medical education is still being inundated with inflating costs and inflating service demands.

Medical education, like other health professions and vocations, has never been financially accepted as an academic venture in this country. From its earliest days, it has operated on a do-it-yourself financial basis. Its origins were in a proprietary mold where it was supposed to make a profit for the entrepreneur physicians who provided the lectures and the preceptorships. Flexner moved the medical schools into the university organization but not into the university budget. It was a marriage of convenience and not of resources. Almost all privately supported universities still insist that the medical school stand on its own financially. In 1968–69, only 2.3 percent of the total operating income of all U.S. medical schools came from the discretionary funds of parent universities. Most of the clinical instruction is still being done by voluntary faculty, and most of the full-time clinical faculty are expected to earn their take through patient care. In no other part of the university are the faculty required to practice what they preach for a fee. Admittedly, there are unique circumstances inherent in the teaching of clinical medicine that produce a reimbursable service and these circumstances have been greatly enhanced by the movement toward universal coverage by third parties. Society should pick up the tab, through private or governmental underwriting, for the cost of the patient services rendered by medical schools but this should not allow the parent university to divorce itself from financial responsibility for medical education.

The financial dichotomy between the parent university and the medical school has produced a direct effect on the medical school's ability to increase their enrollments. While the clinical departments could sell their services as a by-product of their teaching function, the nonclinical departments had no such outside market. The advent of federal traineeships did give them a sort of inside market since those grants provided some general support of departments to which recipient trainees were assigned. In the main, however, the nonclinical departments have been dependent upon budgeted and sponsored funding, and these sources have used graduate education and its correlate, research as the denominator for support. In order to maintain their solvency, therefore, the nonclinical departments have had to put their resources and efforts into graduate education. The result has been a stricture on undergraduate intake and an open house for graduate students.

The factors that have nurtured financially self-sufficient medical education are many and complex. They involve attitudes deeply ingrained in the medical profession, in government, among the public, as well as in universities and medical schools. These attitudes have not only affected the financing of medical schools but have impaired the relationships between medical schools and their parent universities. One can say with more than a little validity that medical education has never been properly assimilated into American universities. The two cannot be expected to hold hands as long as the universities continue to keep their hands tightly in their pockets.

The awkward fit of medical education into academe is responsible for still another major inhibition to its appropriate financing. This stems from the conglomerate of functions and responsibilities of medical education, many of which extend far beyond those usually assigned to universities. Administrators in medical education are well aware of the fact that medical schools are engaged in much more than producing M.D. degrees, that they are the major producers of medical research, patient care, postgraduate and continuing medical education, and a wide spectrum of health science personnel, ranging from doctoral and postdoctoral candidates to technicians. In the middle of this spectrum, small in numbers but large in focus, are the M.D. candidates. It is their small number, however, that is used as the numerator by those who compute the costs of medical education.

Those who administer the medical schools know that M.D.'s are only part of their contribution to health care, but this knowledge does not seem to be shared by the outside world. There is a real lack of financial understanding between those responsible for medical education and those who equate the costs of medical education with the number of M.D.'s produced. This gap is widening as medical schools are handed an ever growing number of assignments beyond the M.D. training and beyond the limits of academe.

This confusing welter of functions and responsibilities means that the public cannot buy an M.D. without buying a total package of training, research, and services. This may be frustrating, but it should not be taken to mean that they are not getting a bargain package—nor one that they do not need. It is obvious that all contents of the package are required by the

Table 1. Sources of operating income to U.S. medical schools * fiscal year 1967–68

	Amount (1,000's)	Percent
Governmental:		
Federal	$ 619,196.	52.7
State and local	172,307	14.6
Total	(791,503.)	(67.3)
Nongovernmental:		
Tuition and fees	48,252.	4.1
Faculty practice funds	48,051.	4.1
Reimbursed services	44,991.	3.8
Support by teaching hospitals	36,694.	3.1
Special project support	128,358.	10.9
Endowment income	35,783.	3.1
Unrestricted gifts	13,590.	1.2
Parent university	27,974.	2.4
Total	(383,893.)	(32.7)
Total all sources	$1,175,396.	(100.0)

* Includes only recorded figures and excludes all income in "kind" such as contributed services of voluntary faculty, free space use, and intangible costs borne by teaching hospitals.
Includes only operating costs and excludes capital cost.
Excludes income for student aid and other expenditures not a part of "production" costs.
(Adapted from data published in Education Number of the *Journal of the American Medical Association*, 210, No. 8, November 24, 1969.)

public and that each would have to be produced elsewhere if medical schools did not provide them. It is equally obvious, even if not recognized, that the means-ends relationships of the various components to each other provide substantial quality and economic values. Most importantly, the aggregate provides the climate essential to the production of the M.D. Medical practice calls as heavily upon the turn-of-mind and the character of the practitioner as it does on his knowledge and skills. Those qualities must be absorbed, even forged, in a structured climate. The research activities of a medical school may not make a direct contribution to the knowledge acquisition of the medical student but their presence helps make his education more than a cookbook experience.

The heavy financial pressures presently being brought upon medical education and the current mood of anti-intellectualism affecting this country hold real dangers for both the quality of medical education and the progress of medical science. The separation of M.D. training from the climate which has nourished its excellence is being advocated by those who are seeking bargain-rate M.D.'s and apparently by institutions seeking a bargain-

Table 2. Sources of facilities construction income to U.S. medical schools,* fiscal year 1968–69

	Amount (1,000's)	Percent
Governmental:		
Federal	$144,893	38.9
State and local	108,011	29.0
Total	(252,904)	(67.9)
Nongovernmental:		
University	70,755	19.0
Contributed	26,817	7.2
Other	21,974	5.9
Total	(119,546)	(32.1)
Total All Sources	$372,450	100.0

* Excludes costs of facilities intended primarily for patient care.

Adapted from data published in Education Number of the *Journal of the American Medical Association*, 210, No. 8, November 24, 1969.

basement entry into the field of medical education. The bargains do not lie in stripped-down models of M.D. training programs but rather in comprehensive packages of medically related functions which permit optimal utilization of resources and provide the stimulus to excellence that the different functions exercise on each other.

The fact that the medical school is a multifunction enterprise, however, creates a responsibility vacuum in its financing, a vacuum that is accentuated because of the expensive nature of each of these functions. One could not assemble a more hagridden set of fiscal resources. Given such a situation, it is not surprising that the various sources of financing tend to outfumble each other in reaching for the medical education bill and to shift their own mounting fiscal difficulties onto each other or onto the medical schools.

Such fiscal buck-passing is inherent in a multiple-function situation where the responsibility for the financing of each function is diverse and categorically defined and where the ends of one serve as the means of another. It is literally true that neither precise costs nor equitable costs of the diverse functions of medical education can be accurately allocated. One hitches on the cost of the other.

Table 1, *Sources of Operating Income to U.S. Medical Schools, Fiscal Year 1967–68,* demonstrates the varied sources underwriting the budgets of medical schools. The problems attendant to the pluralistic financing of

Table 3. Scholarship and loan funds expended by all U.S. medical schools, fiscal year 1968–69

	All schools	Private schools	Public schools
Total enrollment	35,833	16,607	19,226
Loans:			
Funds expended	$21,095,318.	$10,408,074.	$10,687,244.
Number students receiving	20,087	9,057	11,030
Percent of enrollment	56.0	54.5	57.4
Average value per student receiving	$ 1,051.	$ 1,149.	$ 969.
Average value per student enrolled	$ 589.	$ 627.	$ 556.
Scholarships:			
Funds expended	$11,206,305	$ 7,023,321.	$ 4,182,984.
Number students receiving	12,451	6,774	5,677
Percent of enrollment	29.5	40.8	34.7
Average value per student receiving	$ 900.	$ 1,036.	$ 736.
Average value per student enrolled	$ 218.	$ 423.	$ 313.
Loans and scholarships:			
Funds expended	$32,301,623.	$17,431,395.	$14,870,228.
Average value per student enrolled	$ 901.	$ 1,049.	$ 773.

Adapted from data published in Education Number of the *Journal of the American Medical Association*, 210, No. 8, November 24, 1969.

medical education are compounded by the multiple conduits through which funds flow into the budgets of the medical schools. These conduits include general support, project support, student and trainee support, specified activity support, and a variety of special purposes that might fit the interests of donors, foundations, and government at a given time.

In addition, the flow of support is diverted into three separate pools. Funds for operating expenses, construction (Table 2) and student aid (Table 3) are separately metered to the medical school. Even though all may stem from the same source, the appeal for each category must be separately made and separately justified. This means that synchronization of operating needs, facilities needs, and student aid needs is not possible. Since there is no strategy by which the institution can balance its program between the three separate needs, opportunism becomes the controlling principle. The institution must take for each what it can get, from whatever source, and hope the program will balance out.

Much of the blame for the current financial state of medical education can be placed on its administrators and faculties. Medical schools have been guilty of excessive competition with each other and of an obsessive concern with image and status. Each has been more highly concerned with the race for excellence than with the path to excellence. The goal for each has been the sweepstake rather than the daily stakes. This attempt to match the leader across the board has led to proliferation of effort and resources within individual institutions. More importantly, it has failed to produce a basic model for the financing of medical education. How much support is required can be defined only as "more" under current operating policies. This inability to define a satisfactory level of financing has led to a state of frustration on the part of federal and state appropriating bodies and consequent inadequate financing for medical education. It is also leading to bankruptcy on the part of the most highly endowed of the private university medical schools. It is becoming increasingly evident that every medical school cannot be tops in all things and remain solvent and that medical schools must differentiate their programs, both between

Table 4. Cost of medical education computed on various bases, fiscal year 1968–69

Computed on number of medical students divided into total medical school costs	$34,032.
Computed on number of medical students divided into total medical school costs, less research costs	$20,328.
Computed on number of medical students divided into total medical school costs, less research costs and less auxiliary income	$10,461.

Adapted from data published in Education Number of the *Journal of the American Medical Association*, 210, No. 8, November 24, 1969.

institutions and within institutions. This does not mean that medical schools should give up their quest for excellence but rather that they realistically define the starting line and choose more selectively the races they enter.

The lack of clearly defined goals and programs for medical schools can be attributed largely to the nature of medical education financing. The categorical, multiple-source method has not only led to the opportunism noted above, but has forced medical schools to mind their public image more than their programs. To attract funds, they had to attract attention. This attention-oriented programming has been implemented by research pressure on the faculty to publish in professional journals and to earn the professional esteem of their colleagues serving on research funding committees. This concern has tended to shift program and budget control from the medical school administration to the aspirations and funding capabilities of the individual faculty members.

Steps toward sounder financing of medical education

Financing of medical education suffers from lack of a consistent, stable, and organized plan for funding. It is largely dependent upon a variety of separately acting, diverse-interest, and uncommitted sources. Increasingly, much of its responsibilities and its program are far beyond the production of M.D. candidates, and even beyond academic endeavors. Much of the problem of financing medical education is inherent in its nature and can never be fully solved. It could be placed on a more adequate and sounder basis, however, if the following steps were taken:

1. Program budgeting and costing should be adopted in order to identify the separate costs of its varied inseparable responsibilities. This would provide several values:

(*a*) It would permit fixing of the responsibility for financing of each of the responsibilities of the medical school onto the appropriate source of funding;

(*b*) It would enable the medical school to price out the cost of its own aspirations and set priorities on its resources use.

2. A realistic model of the aggregate of activities essential to the education of an M.D. should be developed by medical schools. It is true that there are many activities that must accompany the education of the M.D. if the appropriate climate for his education is to be maintained, and that many of these activities can be best and most economically conducted within the medical school setting. It is equally true, however, that society has a right to support the production of doctors without buying an unrestricted package of other services. If the necessary concept of inseparable services is to be sold, and financing of medical education is to be by the package rather than by the piece, the essential ingredients of the package must be specified. At what level does research cease to be a necessary component of the M.D. educational process and become research for research's sake? At what point does patient care cease to be a by-product of M.D. education and become the product sought? How much graduate education is required to best interact and interfeed with undergraduate medical education? Such questions can be reasonably determined by developing guiding ratios for funding sources. Such ratios would not restrict the medical schools from taking on as much added responsibility as they desired. They would permit society to make choices as to how much it wished to purchase

beyond the basic package while permitting the medical schools the right to say "no" to unfunded and inadvisable demands on its resources.

3. The responsibilities for financing of medical education must be firmly fixed and accepted. All logic points to a federal responsibility for the first-dollar financing of the basic package as defined by the ratios mentioned above. Doctors are considered essential to the national welfare, are treated separately as regards military requirements, and are highly mobile as regards their choice of career location. Also, medical research, health manpower training, and patient care have been accepted as federal responsibilities and have already received substantial federal support. This being the case, it is logical for the basic financing of the medical school to be treated as a function of the federal government. If the annual basic cost could be determined for undergraduate enrollments of various sizes and all medical schools could be reimbursed a high percentage of those costs, it would give each school assurance and continuity for programming and financing. All programs exceeding their component in the basic undergraduate program could then be costed on an incremental basis and funding for them as programs or projects could be sought from federal, state, and private sources.

Basic costs should exclude those for facilities construction and for aid to undergraduate medical students. Construction costs would be figured as a set percentage of basic costs and would be either reserved for payment of interest and capital on borrowed funds or used for replacement and modernization. Future federal grants for construction would be restricted to facilities for research, for special programs outside basic undergraduate medical education, and for increased enrollment of undergraduates. Tuition rates would be determined and retained by each school, but one-third of all tuition received would be used for student aid. Based on 1968–69 tuition charges, this would have provided about $16 million for scholarships as compared with the approximately $11.2 million that were actually provided to students. No federal scholarship funds would be provided under this plan, but federal loans would be continued. Both facilities and student aid funds would be augmented from whatever other sources each school might be able to find.

Costs directly associated with patient care would not be included in the basic costs, but a clinical teaching component for both faculty and house staff would be included. The affiliated hospital would exclude any such teaching component from its third-party reimbursable costs, but aside from that, would seek full reimbursement from patients and third parties for the cost of all services rendered, including the patient care actually provided by faculty and house staff.

The cost to the federal government of such a plan for funding the front-dollar costs of undergraduate medical education can be determined only after a decision is made as to the elements to be included and the percentage to be funded. Assuming a federal share of one-half the basic costs, a general estimate would be in the area of about $250 million, or about $6,000 per undergraduate student in fiscal 1972 for the basic program and, using a 10 percent factor, $25 million for facilities reserve, or a total of $275 million. This total would equal about 50 percent of the regular operating budgets of American medical schools during 1972.

This basic program approach permits a four-layer arrangement for federal support of medical schools. The first layer would be the basic program support and facilities replacement annual capitation payment. This would provide support for those instructional, research, and graduate education costs considered necessary and inseparable for a balanced undergraduate education program, and would represent the "first dollars" in the medical school budget.

The second layer would be special purpose support for such special orientation of the basic program as federal policy might indicate from time to time. This support would also be on a capitation basis and would augment the basic program support. Such special purposes might include added enrollment, minority student enrollment, subeconomic student enrollment, speed-up student enrollment, etc.

The third layer would be project support and would be paid on a project budget basis. It would include project research, demonstration teaching and patient care projects, community service, etc.

The fourth layer would include allied health personnel training programs and those graduate degree programs in excess of their ratios in the basic program. These would be supported on a per capita rate to be negotiated for three-year periods with the individual institution.

This arrangement for financing would mean that the basic program support represented federal responsibility for the "first dollars" in the medical school budget. It would insure that any cutbacks in federal support of medical schools, due either to stringencies in the federal budget or to changes in federal policy direction, would affect the ongoing medical school program last. It would also permit competition between medical schools for special support for special excellence.

Neither the numbers nor the design of the above plan of financing are overly important. The crucial need is for acceptance by the federal government of responsibility for the front-end financing of medical education. It has accepted the responsibility for adequate health care of every individual. It now has the obligation to assure the necessary medical manpower to meet that commitment. Such assurance requires predictable, continuous front end financial support of medical education. Such basic support to all medical schools would serve to increase and expand the initiative of the medical schools in their search for excellence beyond the level that the federal government can financially or politically support. Medical schools have demonstrated a capacity to find a variety of sources of funds and should be encouraged to aggressively exploit them. The time has come, however, when the cracks between these sources have widened too greatly to permit adequate, consistent and orderly funding of medical education.

Author's recommendations

1. The federal government should accept ultimate major responsibility for financing medical education. This responsibility should be firmly fixed and accepted and include the cost of both facilities and student aid.

2. Medical education financing must be based on a consistent, stable and organized plan which would include:

   a) Program budgeting and costing to fix responsibilities for financing and enable medical schools to price out the cost of their own aspirations and set priorities on resources;

   b) Development by medical schools of a realistic model of the aggregate of activities essential to the education of an M.D.

Coauthors' comments

Dr. Anlyan:

The medical schools of the United States are a national resource. What should be the federal government's share of the basic support of medical schools? What is the best method of support?

Whereas exact data on the true cost per year per medical student is lacking, it is estimated that the range is between $16,000–$25,000 exclusive of sponsored research and the operating costs of the teaching hospital. If this figure of $16,000–$25,000 per student per year is accepted, then the position of the Association of American Medical Colleges * suggesting basic federal support of $5,000 per student per year would represent from one-third to one-fifth as the federal share. The Carnegie Commission has proposed $4,000 per student per year. Current legislation before Congress

* "AAMC Program for the Expansion of Medical Education." *J. Med. Educ.* 46: 105–115, Feb. 1971.

includes a capitation provision for $2,500 per student per year for the first three years and $4,000 for the year of graduation. My personal view is that the level of $5,000 per student per year should be viewed as an absolute minimum.

The approach described above is the "capitation" system. Obviously one needs "caputs" to "capitate" and the heads will belong to the medical students. The capitation system also represents the "first dollar" approach in contrast to the "last dollar" approach. The latter is undesirable since it advocates making up the "last dollars" that a medical school needs to balance its books. The liabilities of the last dollar approach also include the inability of the medical school to plan ahead and the removal of incentives to seek private and state support ("Let's leave it to Uncle Sam"). In due time all the medical schools would look alike.

In contrast, the "first dollar" approach would give dependable and predictable basic support. Private and state support would be additive with the incentive that every additional dollar would enable the school to move into areas of excellence above the common national denominator.

The capitation approach can also be used for a second layer of support for special incentives to achieve national goals, e.g., increase in enrollment and increase in minority students. These incentives should be special bonuses and not tied into the basic capitation support. Otherwise the downward spiral into the maelstrom of bankruptcy will never be reversed.

Additional federal support should be available for innovations in medical education. Since innovation is not "capitatable," it should be based on a project application mechanism with peer review. Innovations should not only include changes in the fundamental content of components of the continuum of medical education but also the introduction of learners into new health care systems such as health maintenance organizations.

Finally, great caution must be exercised to avoid "robbing Peter" (the research dollar) in "paying Paul" (the education dollar). Both forms of support are fundamental to the role of the academic medical centers of the nation as national resources for the health care system.

Dr. Beck:

With the import of increasingly tight budgets, those of us concerned with the future planning of health sciences centers in North America have been confronted with a dilemma. Do we foster comparable and stereotyped facilities throughout or do we allow the development of special capabilities or resources as part of an overall plan for a variety of excellent centers as a national resource available to all? Because of this dilemma, decisions on desirable major projects are being deferred. Although it may be possible to initiate these at this time, we cannot be certain that it will be possible to carry them through without an assurance of reasonable growth in our budgets. In my view, the establishment of a policy of selectivity and concentration is urgent, and this inevitably demands preferential support for first-rate health science (and I use this term in its broadest sense) at the right places. In making these selections we must rely on the advice of the best experts in science, education, and government, using the well established and generally proven principle of peer review. These experts should be charged with selecting genuinely promising, as distinct from fashionable, fields for special encouragement, not simply to fill a local or regional need but to meet an identified national one.

We in North America must begin to accept publicly what an increasing number of scientists, educators, and politicians recognize privately, that not all of our health science and allied health facilities can be equally good or competent at everything. We must concentrate on support to meet national objectives, and this will lead to a select number of university health science centers that are strong in specified areas. Inevitably, those less favored will not have an equal opportunity to achieve excellence except in the event that the selected areas prove to be essential to every center. Although we cannot feel altogether happy with this prospect, the alternative is to spread our limited resources too thinly to be effective anywhere. A corollary to this view dictates a reevaluation of presently established programs. Whereas there is excellent sense in allowing certain centers to be self-perpetuating, we show very bad judgment if we hesitate to close down centers when the national need dictates and the claims of others prove stronger. Such a policy requires courage and the cooperation of the universities, since they must develop their own individual priorities which may put an end to some projects to make way for fresh new lines of research.

It follows that not every university should build up specialist teaching and research facilities in every subject area. This would create an even greater concentration of resources in certain fields and would force the adoption of policies favoring regionalization of these facilities in "a multi-university concept," using this term in a new sense. Such a regionalization of resources ought to be the product of selective growth that minimizes the impact of selective termination and provides for easier transfers of students and faculty between institutions.

Dr. Medearis:

Cost to the student. It seems to me that the support of medical students, their tuition, board, room and various expenses, has not received sufficient attention in this chapter on the financing of medical education. Federal and state governments, foundations, and educational institutions have all been concerned by this serious problem, but none has sufficiently addressed it. We must answer the question of whether the expense of the education of the medical student will be made free to him and this cost will be borne by other elements of society, or, whether the student will, through a tuition and loan program, support all or some of it.

It seems to me that medical education is clearly of great financial benefit to those who receive it, and therefore that the student who can should pay for some of its cost. At the same time medical education is of great benefit to the entirety of society and its direct benefits are received by a population much larger than the medical students who directly participate. Accordingly, the cost to the student of obtaining a medical education should not be borne entirely by federal or state governments; at the same time the medical student should directly fund a portion of his education because he is going to receive an economic benefit far greater than that which he will contribute. Thus, I believe the approach expressed by Professor Zaccharis and programs like that recently begun at Yale, Duke, and the Ford Foundation deserve serious consideration.

The concept of first-dollar support. Dr. Anlyan has most appropriately and emphatically stressed the absolute need that federal support of medical education be first-dollar support. The purpose of this comment is to emphasize that this federal support must be such that state support is not lost. States receive direct and great benefit from their medical schools and their support of them must be substantial and it must not be solely deficit-correcting in nature. Medical education cannot serve society better until there is stability in medical educational funding. Medical educators must recognize the need to and then provide the means by which we can justify federal first-dollar support, and state support through a process of public disclosure and accountability.

Unless federal support becomes first-dollar support and state support continues strong (and becomes stronger), private giving, both individual and foundation, probably will decrease, if not cease. Income from private sources should provide a margin for excellence. The ability of the institution to innovate, to create new programs; to experiment in teaching and organizational techniques, to meet unforeseen needs in a flexible and effective manner, and to pursue, find, and create new information and new knowledge must be ensured; to a significant extent many medical schools depend on private funds for this. Private funds must not be used to provide first-dollar support for medical education. Moreover, this income represents the measure of the ability of private individuals and foundations to assume part of the responsibility for educating physicians. If for every dollar the university attracted from the private sector of the economy a dollar of state support or a dollar of federal support were to be removed, the incentive for private giving would be lost and the support from that source would cease. Both state and federal governments have urged universities to assume the greatest possible responsibility for their financial destiny. However, if the schools are to carry out this mandate they should not be penalized for their success. Thus, federal (and state if possible) support should be first-dollar support, not last-dollar, deficit, make-up support.

Dr. Van der Kloot:

One of the most misunderstood aspects of medical school financing is the allocation of faculty time and the factors determining faculty size. For cost billing, faculty time has been sorted into four categories: teaching, service, administration, and research. When keeping his time sheet, the professor totals up the hours in the classroom, adds the time spent directly preparing for teaching, the hours at the bedside, and the time spent with committees and the like. All remaining time is then charged to research. These calculations usually show that only one-fifth of the time is spent with teaching; the bulk goes to research.

This is very misleading. The time allocated for research almost invariably includes all time spent in the library, at seminars, talking with one's colleagues, and at scientific meetings. If I were to stop research tomorrow, all of these activities must still be done, otherwise I would soon lose all touch with my field and all effectiveness as a teacher. In the sciences, a professor must devote the greater fraction of his time to simply keeping up with his specialty. Reasonable time-effort studies would add this category to the choices and would thereby put to rest the fancy that inordinate time goes to research. Faculty research must be encouraged because, among other things, it is powerful incentive toward keeping up with rapidly moving fields. It is a commonplace observation that professors who give up research rarely retain the intense drive and self-discipline needed to keep up with the information explosion.

There is another aspect of faculty organization that is difficult for laymen to appreciate; it is best illustrated by example. Suppose that I wanted to get an accurate picture of how a muscle works. If I go to the library I can find out a great deal, but all the information in text books and review articles is inevitably several years old, and hundreds of papers have been published in the meantime. My best course is to talk with my colleague who is interested in this field. He is constantly reading the latest papers, evaluating their methods and conclusions, and incorporating them into his picture of muscle function. In a real sense our knowledge of muscle is stored in the heads of a few hundred professors.

The modern medical school can be understood only when the role of professor in processing, ordering, and storing information is taken into account. The pressure for increasing faculty size comes from the exploding supply of information. One hundred years ago one professor could store and process all important information in physiology; now a department of fifteen or twenty may seem inadequate for the task. Department size is determined more by the breadth of knowledge that must be handled than by the number of students that must be taught. Great universities are marked by a broad breadth of faculty interests. In every major area of knowledge there is a professor who is an outstanding authority. Since significant advances in science often depend upon taking ideas from one field and applying them to another, scholars compete for the chance to join universities at which they can receive this kind of intellectual backup. And a significant fraction of faculty time is spent teaching other faculty members. In the best medical schools, for example, the basic science faculty plays a major role in the continuing education of the clinical faculty. Consequently scientific faculties will always be pressing for expansion in numbers and in faculty quality.

The view that the university is solely responsible for teaching, merely as an extension of the high school, is one of the most potentially disastrous ideas circulating in our society. The university has traditionally been responsible for teaching, for research, and for the preservation of knowledge. The tradition evolved because each activity feeds on the others. Any attempt to evaluate how well the job is being done by measuring only one parameter is bound to be incredibly misleading.

References

1. U.S. Department of Health, Education, and Welfare Staff Task Force for Health Manpower, *Manpower for Health: National Needs and Federal Programs.* Washington, D.C.: U.S. Government Printing Office, July, 1969.
2. Carnegie Commission on Higher Education, *A Special Report and Recommendations.* New York: Carnegie Corporation, Dec. 1968.